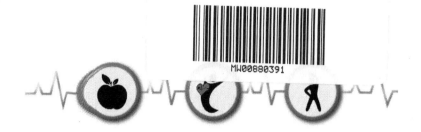

DAILY
INSPIRATIONS FOR
EATING AND
TRAINING
SUCCESS
365

A Simple Day by Day Program to Redefine Your Healthy Self

JILL KOEGEL, RD, CSSD, CDE

D.I.E.T.S. 365
Daily Inspirations for Eating and Training Success

ISBN: 978-1724788252

Copyright © 2018 by Jill R. Koegel

cnomaha@gmail.com
www.certifiednutritionomaha.com

Design & layout by Lighthouse24

Introduction

If you want to lose weight, you can do it in hundreds of ways and get varied results. But if your goal is getting healthy, you will need to commit to making changes that will stick. As these changes become easier, they will begin to make a cumulative difference in your health. You will achieve the frame of mind necessary for lifelong healthy success.

"Jan" was a client in my practice who needed a mixture of solutions to her various health problems. She continued to tell me of her constant struggles and her need for daily support. Jan committed to review and tackle her goals every day to stay on track. D.I.E.T.S. 365 was born out of this very real and human need for structure and direction in everyday life. The approach is simple and might seem obvious to the experienced dieter, but the concepts are proven to be challenging to prioritize in everyday life.

A simplified approach to healthy lifestyles allows small successes in a life full of other priorities. To think "one step at a time" is a sure way to achieve goals, especially when overwhelmed. I dedicate this book to my clients, who have taught me perspective and offered me the experience to help others succeed.

How to Use this Book

Should you start at the beginning of this book? If today is January 1st the answer is yes! If it's not, start at today's date. If this is your first try at healthy changes, follow the calendar in order. If you've read other books to improve your lifestyle, you might be more likely to skip around. The most important part: make each task a priority.

D.I.E.T.S. 365 was designed to inspire you through an entire year. You can read it from January to December, or skip around. Notice there are actually 366 D.I.E.T.S. in case of a leap year! Make note of the days that help you the most, and read them over and over. You'll notice that each D.I.E.T. falls into one of three categories: Food, Fitness, or Wellness. If you prefer, you can choose a reading from the category that serves you best on any particular day.

FOOD

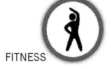
FITNESS

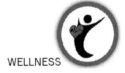
WELLNESS

I suggest reading your entry first thing in the morning or read the following day when you go to bed, so you are prepared to take action when you wake up! No matter how you decide to do it, you will see how working on one task at a time helps you achieve quick mini success. By focusing on daily goals you will build your foundation, experience heightened awareness, and develop lifelong habits.

January 1

Each time you start something new there is fresh curiosity about it, but there might also be judgment about what was done before and what didn't work. Today, focus on the newness of a clean slate.

Today is the first day of a new approach, using a specific strategy each day to guide you. As you read, interpret, and apply messages, be aware that your process will likely be different from the next person. The application of D.I.E.T.S. 365 in your life will be unique and tailored to you. While focusing on your own goals, avoid outside influences that may deter you.

D.I.E.T. #1

Turn away from judgments of your own, and from anyone else. Any time a negative thought creeps in, remind yourself that this new journey belongs to you. It is time for you to succeed, each and every day.

January 2

Pick one thing. It's the premise of D.I.E.T.S 365, and it's a strategy you can return to if you happen to get off track. Dog ear the page, or remember... just one thing. It's simple to accomplish one thing when you have a plan to do it.

It could be drinking an extra glass of water at lunch, or taking a walk after dinner. Prepare yourself to achieve your "thing," and make sure it is realistic and appropriate. Don't pick going for a walk after dinner if the forecast calls for rain, unless you have a treadmill!

You will see specific suggestions in the coming days and months, but for now, practice by choose *anything* that makes sense for your goals.

D.I.E.T. #2

Start the habit of picking one daily goal to focus on. Now, close your eyes, think of your goal, and picture yourself following through.

January 3

After the holidays, there are leftovers galore! Goodies from neighbors, remnants from work parties, and drinks in the fridge. Take today to clean out the pantry, and clear off the countertops. Remember, what remains will likely be eaten. Put aside any feelings of being wasteful, and instead, be mindful of your waist!

If you have items that are unopened, consider donating them to a local charity, your church, or somewhere it can go to better use! If you don't donate it, realize that wasting your goodies is healthier than consuming them, so go ahead and fill up the dumpster. This is one of the best ways to start "clean" for the New Year.

D.I.E.T. #3

Purge your leftovers. Remove temptations to avoid procrastination of your health goals! Access to them is an invitation to fail, especially early in the year when you are trying to get started on your health goals.

January 4

Eating late into the night is unhealthy for many reasons. The body isn't created to utilize calories late in the day as well as early in the day. If you eat close to bedtime, you will train your body to store calories, and you will be less likely to enjoy quality sleep.

Choose a time to stop. It might depend on the time you go to bed, but typically allow a three to four hour window between dinnertime and lights out. If you already have this habit, you might consider a change such as eating your last meal earlier. Have a light dinner and stop eating for the night. You don't have to make this an "all of the time" rule, but do it today. Plan something to do that will distract you, or plan to go to bed a little earlier. This pattern can improve your overall energy quickly, so give it a try.

D.I.E.T. #4

Stop eating after a light dinner. Give your body a break from digesting and absorbing food. Think of it as a "fast," if that helps you stick to it.

January 5

Have a cup of water upon reading this entry. Eight to sixteen ounces will help refresh and hydrate you, give you a boost of energy, and help move your bowels! Focus on drinking more water today than usual. You might fill a reusable bottle before leaving the house, or order water with your lunch.

Besides its hydrating effect, drinking a warm cup of water with lemon can also be an appetite suppressant and a digestive aid. However you do it, add water, and make it more than your typical hydration habits. Note how your energy level improves!

D.I.E.T. #5

Focus on hydration. You can drink other fluids too, but make sure you consume at least half your body weight in ounces of water. If you are considered obese, add your current weight and your desired weight. Divide by two, and drink half of this adjusted body weight in ounces of water.

January 6

When you go to the store, do you spend most of your time in the produce section? If not, it's a great habit to start! When you get home, clean and store fruits and veggies where they are easily accessed. Remember to slide older items forward so you waste as little as possible!

Don't just think about steamed veggies as side dishes, but remember that raw veggies, prepped ahead of time provide a quick, satisfying snack. Mushrooms, peppers, cherry tomatoes, and cucumbers are great for munching! Use a calendar or menu planner to write down how and when you will eat your fresh items.

D.I.E.T. #6

Make produce more usable by purchasing, cleaning, and chopping ahead of time. Then, make it more accessible by putting produce in clear containers in the front of your fridge. Take a picture and remember how it makes you feel to have fresh, healthy snacks and meal items on hand.

January 7

Choose an earlier bedtime, even if just for tonight. It is proven that people who go to bed earlier and get up earlier are more productive. Hitting the pillow fifteen minutes ahead and getting up fifteen minutes earlier is the same total amount of sleep, but it can make a huge difference. Remember that a bit less TV time at night means more relaxing quiet time in the morning.

It isn't as easy as it seems, but remind yourself of the benefits this fifteen-minute change will provide. You are less apt to watch television in the morning versus the evening, so you can get something much more worthwhile accomplished. For example, truly enjoy sipping a warm cup of tea or coffee, instead of drinking it in the car or spilling it on your way out the door!

D.I.E.T. #7

Set your alarm fifteen minutes early and plan to enjoy the sunrise, read your next D.I.E.T., take a walk, or just pay attention to the peace and quiet.

January 8

Eat breakfast. Prepare something ahead of time, or plan what you will make. Include protein, whole grain carbs, and a source of healthy fats if possible. An example for today is an egg on whole grain toast with avocado. If you'd rather make something ahead, you can prepare "overnight oats" with equal portions of oats, milk, and yogurt. Add nuts, seeds, chopped fruit, or flavorings such as vanilla extract or cinnamon, if desired. Mix together and soak in the refrigerator overnight.

If you already eat breakfast, change it up and make sure you include as much protein as possible. Studies show that eating more protein in the morning helps prevent cravings later in the day. My favorite breakfast proteins include eggs, protein smoothies, nutty granola atop Greek yogurt, and chicken sausage.

D.I.E.T. #8

Plan or enjoy a balanced breakfast and notice how it affects your cravings and choices later in the day.

January 9

Changing your environment can be as easy as setting the table. Some people find that setting the table also commits them to eating at home. You can even do it before you leave for the day! If you don't normally sit down to a meal in the evening, this will be enough of a change. If you do, try setting your table in a new way to enhance your eating experience.

Adding color to the table by using placemats or different colored dishware can encourage healthier choices. Brighten the room by adding a tablecloth or placing a centerpiece on the table. It doesn't have to be flowers, as a fruit bowl or a child's artwork can liven things up too! Wrap silverware in napkins, or watch a video to learn how to fold napkins in a fancy way.

D.I.E.T. #9

Set your table differently. My mom is the master of tabletops, and it's always fun to see what she's come up with for a centerpiece! See if it changes your thoughts about staying home for dinner.

January 10

Ever think you're hungry, but then realize you're actually bored? It's common for people to eat for reasons other than hunger. The urge to eat is often brought on by emotions, and by the time a person realizes it, the damage of a heavy snack or meal is already done.

Today, use a hunger scale to bring mindfulness to your reasons for eating. A rating of "1" means you are physically feeling symptoms of extreme hunger, and a rating of "10" means you are uncomfortably full. Recognize your hunger and whether using a hunger scale causes you to make better choices. This is a practice in mindfulness and can be a great place to return to, any day of the year!

D.I.E.T. #10

Rate your hunger before you eat any snack or meal. Make sure you are between 1 and 5 before starting, and if not, determine a new action to take that doesn't involve food. Note: To avoid overeating, try not to reach a hunger rating of "1."

January 11

A bathroom scale can be a useless tool, especially when you are just starting out. There are a variety of inaccuracies that could easily derail you. To improve accuracy, make sure your scale has fresh batteries, weigh yourself without clothes first thing in the morning, and empty your bladder before you step on. Even after all of these steps, fluctuations in weight are common, and can be hard to explain.

Instead of weighing every day, leave your scale in a closet and get it out once a week or less. This will allow you to see a trend and the accumulation of your efforts. It also keeps you guessing and working as hard as you can to see that weekly success!

D.I.E.T. #11

Put the scale away. Even though a small weight loss can propel you forward, a small weight gain could be a catastrophe to your confidence.

January 12

Follow a Mediterranean-style eating plan today. Known for its benefits of lowering cholesterol and being heart healthy, it is also great for the mind, as it has been shown to be helpful in slowing cognitive decline.

This way of eating can easily become a new lifestyle, because it is full of delicious and colorful foods. The foods to focus on including are lean proteins, particularly fish and plant based proteins, brightly colored vegetables, healthy fats such as olive oil and nuts, and whole grains. You may have to take a trip to the store, but the foods you need to purchase are simple and readily available.

D.I.E.T. #12

Have avocado with your whole grain toast in the morning, walnuts for a morning snack, a big salad with olive oil based dressing for lunch, and grilled salmon with quinoa for dinner. Snack on lower sugar Greek yogurt and berries in the afternoon. A basic Mediterranean-style day is simple, fresh, and healthy!

January 13

Strength training is important in overall body metabolism. The more muscle you create, the faster your body turns calories into energy instead of storing fat them as fat. There are simple things you can do to incorporate strength training, no matter your age or ability level.

Choose a few muscle groups to challenge. For example, the chest group can be worked with pushups, planks, or bench press, and you don't even need equipment. Try sets of squats, or walk up and down stairs to challenge your legs. Shoulder presses, bicep curls, and triceps extension are simple exercises to finish your routine. Spend at least ten minutes on at least three exercises. If you are more experienced, try a circuit of various moves for a full body workout. Write down what you did so you can repeat it!

D.I.E.T. #13

Incorporate strength training. It can be an energizing step to take, and it is sure to leave you feeling empowered.

January 14

It is easy to make an unhealthy eating choice when faced with a limited menu, or when surrounded by people enjoying fried foods and sugary drinks. Eating at home or from home is a helpful goal if you are tempted to overeat or choose fries over steamed broccoli.

Making a lunch to take to the office and creating a quick and delicious dinner at home isn't as hard as it seems. Keep it simple! Grab a serving of almonds, a piece of fruit, a string cheese and a protein shake and your lunch is done. It doesn't have to be a sandwich or fancy salad, but those are great choices too. For dinner, chop some grilled chicken and serve over a large spinach salad. Add hard-boiled eggs, shredded cheese, and lots of extra veggies. Top with an oil based dressing.

D.I.E.T. #14

Eat at home today. You can eat it on the run if needed, but choose foods only from your kitchen.

January 15

Do you know how much you are eating? While calories are probably not the most important thing when compared to nutritional quality, consistent overeating will most definitely result in weight gain. Keep in mind, the serving sizes you need may be very different from your spouse, friend, or child, but a helpful goal when trying to lose weight is to decrease the portions you are currently eating.

While serving sizes on labels are not always appropriate for everyone, awareness of how much you are eating is one of the keys to long-term success. In order to be honest with yourself, it is important to first be knowledgeable about how much your food weighs, and to learn how to visualize a smaller portion.

D.I.E.T. #15

Use a food scale today. Measure any food that is not whole. Be sure to measure snacks such as almonds and crackers, and compare proteins such as pre-cooked versus cooked meats.

January 16

Today, change how you are spending time. Here are some ideas to get you started:

- Complete a seated meditation for at least ten minutes, instead of checking social media. Use an app if you prefer a guided experience.
- Take a walk for the majority of your lunch break. Have a quick meal with the time remaining!
- Go to the store after work, instead of through the drive through.
- Visit your favorite healthy blog or search a new one, instead of watching television.
- Plan a way to get to bed thirty minutes early, instead of watching the news.
- Pack your lunch for tomorrow, instead of having an evening snack.

D.I.E.T. #16

Decide on a part of your day to insert one healthy change. This is proof that you have time, or can make time for new habits!

January 17

It isn't a bad thing to feel hungry. Physical hunger, when coupled with shakiness, nervousness, or dizziness definitely deserves attention, but a growling stomach doesn't necessarily require feeding. If hunger is interfering with your day, have a protein rich or healthy fat based snack and move on. If it is just a rumble in your stomach, or a boss who stressed you out, try to go hungry!

Remember that you will eat again soon, and that skipping an emotionally driven snack will actually help you manage those emotions in the long run. Instead of eating, write down what you are feeling in a journal, take a few deep breaths, or talk to someone trustworthy.

D.I.E.T. #17

Let your body feel hungry, and notice that you can work through it. A loud stomach will quiet down if you wait a little while, and it is encouraging to be able to sit through some physical and/or emotional hunger.

January 18

Dry skin, hair, and nails are common during the winter months. The air is dry and the temperatures are colder, and winter naturally decreases the thirst mechanism. For all these reasons hydrating with plenty of water is hard, but helpful.

Coffee, tea, and other warm drinks are soothing and comforting, especially when it's cold. There is nothing wrong with a warm drink, including a caffeinated choice, but they often take the place of water. If you get headaches trying to avoid caffeine, it may be a cue that you need more water in your day. If you have a caffeine habit, you may need to ease into it, but keeping this page marked and working to gradually exchange water for other beverages will be an amazing achievement.

D.I.E.T. #18

Drink only water today. It's a tough one for many people, but this goal will get you focused and energized again.

January 19

There are many gadgets that can help you measure "steps," and wearing a device that tracks your every move can be a great accountability tool! Many studies show that sedentary lifestyles are more risky than any behavior or bad habit. If you could do one thing to tackle many areas of health, it would be to move more.

If you don't have a pedometer, tracking device or fancy watch, don't worry! Moving more can mean purposefully parking in a new spot at work, or walking up an extra flight of stairs and back down to where you were going. It means adding something you wouldn't normally do. If you have a job that is mostly seated, set your watch or another timer to alert you on the hour, and simply get up from a seated position.

D.I.E.T. #19

Add steps today. This could mean 1,000 extra steps on your tracking device, or it could be two or three additional moving opportunities added to your day.

January 20

Accountability is critical in your efforts to improve your health. If you are your own best critic, it can be helpful for accountability. You likely hold yourself to a high standard. However, if you are like most people, you may need a little nudge to be more mindful of what you are eating.

To determine what kind of changes need to be made, record what you are eating. What we are actually eating isn't always the same portion and item we remember eating. If you write it down when you eat it, you can be more accurate as to what you are actually consuming so that you can improve it. This awareness is key, and in addition to simply knowing what is going in, the fact that you are recording it will affect your choices today!

D.I.E.T. #20

Journal today. Write down what you eat, when you eat it. It can be handwritten in a notebook, entered in an app, or recorded in the notes on your phone. Don't judge yourself, but be honest so you can notice patterns and habits that need improvement.

January 21

Boredom is usually acted upon. Once you determine you are bored, you typically do something about it. Do you call a friend, fold laundry, or get on the computer? It's much more fun to explore the pantry, isn't it? Boredom can certainly cause overeating, and it can lead to a lifestyle of eating for reasons other than hunger.

Many people tell me they don't even know how it feels to be hungry because they graze all day long. Usually this is a form of coping, procrastination, or entertainment. Today, create a list of things you will do to avoid becoming bored. These could include: starting a load of laundry, writing a grocery list, preparing fresh produce, vacuuming, or cleaning a toilet. I know, cleaning a toilet may sound like the last thing you would want to do, but *doing* something is the key to forgetting about food when you are bored.

D.I.E.T. #21

Combat boredom! Make a list of action steps, and follow them if you get "hungry" for something to do.

January 22

You may have tried low carb, low fat, low calorie or high protein. Focusing on what to include versus what to avoid is a more positive and helpful way to stay on track.

Healthy fats lower cholesterol, provide satiety, and help control blood sugars. They are an example of what to include! Fats can be polyunsaturated such as omega three fatty acids, and monounsaturated fats. To increase the ratio of healthy fats in your diet, eat a serving of nuts today, such as walnuts or almonds. One serving is one ounce, or about a medium-sized handful. You can also try them as nut butters. If you can't eat nuts, try chia or ground flax seeds. Add a tablespoon of olive oil in cooking, or over a green salad. A three-ounce serving of salmon or fresh tuna can also provide adequate heart healthy fats. Avocados are another one of my favorites, if you prefer a plant-based choice.

D.I.E.T. #22

There are many ways to add healthy fats to your diet. Include them today, and notice how they fill you up with long lasting energy.

January 23

Getting "stuck in a rut" can lead to giving in or giving up, so prevent it by being creative and perhaps a bit adventurous with your meals. One way to do this is to find a new recipe and head to the store for any necessary groceries. Then, plan when you will prepare and serve it!

Search the Internet, check social media, or dig into your grandmother's old cookbook. Or head to the store, browse the magazine section, select a recipe, and get your groceries all in one stop. Look for an idea that expands your horizons. Go out on a limb with something you don't normally cook at home, like tofu or salmon. You can also choose a side dish that changes up your meal, such as a new vegetable or quinoa.

D.I.E.T. #23

Try a new recipe today. This gets the creative juices flowing, and it gives you the confidence that you can cook at home. If you have extras, freeze or refrigerate leftovers in portion-controlled containers. Start a "new recipes" file and store the ones you like for future use.

January 24

Caring for something other than ourselves can be an experience full of love. Typically, you get much more out of caring for a pet than what you put in, which isn't always the case with humans! Besides the love, distractions, and smiles, pets offer accountability when it comes to taking walks or playing in the yard. Take advantage of their ability to help you with your health!

If you aren't an animal lover, caring for plants or working around your home can also reap many benefits. An obvious result is increased calorie burn due to the physical activity required. Another benefit from gardening and doing yard work is stress reduction. Perhaps most fulfilling is the sense of accomplishment felt in finishing a project, or in beautifying your yard.

D.I.E.T. #24

Give extra attention to your pets and plants today. You will be rewarded for your efforts.

January 25

Controlling portions is a great way to lose weight, and it can be a relatively simple approach. Even if you don't have a weight problem, overeating is hard on your body. The serving sizes on a package aren't always what you should consume, but they are a good place to start when trying to reduce portions. The trick is to also listen to your hunger and aim to eat for physical, rather than emotional reasons.

To encourage proper portions, place measuring tools inside packaged foods. Small scoops, plastic ramekins, or measuring cups work great. Even if your item isn't open yet, you can place these inside the box for when you are ready to open the packaging. Or, place them in your cupboard, next to bags of unopened items.

D.I.E.T. #25

Place one to 2 ounce ramekins, or small measuring cups inside packaged foods. It's great to avoid purchasing packaged items at all, but if you do, practice portion control.

January 26

The health benefits of tea are numerous. The more stress you endure with the demands of everyday life, the more damage you do to your body on a microscopic level. Consuming antioxidants can help reverse some of the damage. Both black and green teas top the lists of foods with the highest concentration of a large class of antioxidants called polyphenols.

Appetite suppression is another benefit for those who choose green tea, due to its ability to stabilize blood sugars. In addition, drinking a decaf version helps hydration status. Choosing tea can be therapeutic in these ways, but it can also help you avoid other actions you might take, or drinks you might reach for.

D.I.E.T. #26

Drink tea today. If you're looking for something soothing, try it warm or hot. If it is refreshment and overall boost you're craving, have it iced. Try the regular version with a tea bag, explore Matcha, or try another powdered or loose tea varieties.

January 27

Feeding someone else can be satisfying and comforting. Invite a health-conscious friend or couple for dinner. Choose people who are on a healthy journey, or who can support you. You might also offer this to your spouse as a special "date." Think of your guest's needs, likes, and goals, and aim to accomplish them alongside him/her.

Need suggestions for what to prepare? Keep it simple! Plan a vegetable tray with a healthy dip such as hummus or guacamole for pre-dinner munching. Prepare a salad ahead of time with a simple oil and vinegar based dressing. For the entrée, grilled fish or chicken is always simple, or search for a meatless option such as lentil sloppy Joes or homemade veggie burgers. Skip dessert, or offer berries with fresh whipped cream.

D.I.E.T. #27

Offer a meal. You will gain support from your invitee, and you will gain confidence in your ability to serve a healthy meal.

January 28

Maybe I focus on the color green during the winter because I miss the lush green lawns and leaves that have been gone for what seems like an eternity! Let green foods be an appropriate substitute today! They offer tons of nutrients for a relatively small calorie cost.

Think salads or be more creative, but typically green foods are vegetables, so this is my sneaky way of getting more veggies into your diet. You don't have to use the ideas below, but they are examples of how to increase your intake of nutrients and fiber. Green might just become your favorite color!

D.I.E.T. #28

Focus on the color green. Think green for every meal. Spread avocado on toast, and have kiwi for a morning snack. Include a giant salad with colorful greens at lunch. Include cucumber, green pepper, and bright leafy salad greens.
Have green tea in the afternoon and include steamed broccoli, beans, kale, or spinach for dinner.

January 29

Creating a stronger core is important for anyone on a healthy journey. Preventing injury and becoming better at movement should be the main goal. One of the best exercises for the core is the plank, of which there are many modifications. Perform a wall version if this is your first time:

To begin, face the wall. Step away so you can place your forearms and palms flat on the wall, fingertips pointing up. Place your elbows at shoulder level. You should be looking slightly down. If your hips sag toward the wall, pull your belly button in, as though you are "sucking in" to zip up your pants. Bring your hips in a line with the back of your head, and straighten your legs to be in that same line. Try to flatten the heels on the floor. Breathe. Hold this position as long as you can, rest, and repeat. If it's too easy, try it on the floor, elbows below shoulders, pulling your abdominals in and upward.

D.I.E.T. #29

Do three planks, holding each as long as possible. Try three in a row, with a bit of rest between, or do one in the morning, one at lunch, and one before bed.

January 30

Trying to get people to eat more veggies is hard, unless you teach them how to *like* more veggies! There are ways to sneak more vegetables in, such as by using purees in casseroles or by spreading them on pizza

Try seasoning them differently, using infused oils and herbs like rosemary and garlic. Consider new cooking methods. Roasted and grilled vegetables take on an entirely different taste, and are easy to prepare. Try different tools to chop, slice, rice, and dice your veggies differently. Consider purchasing a spiralizer to make noodle shapes with vegetables such as zucchini and sweet potatoes. These aren't exactly noodles, but they are fun and tasty. If you like spaghetti squash, you don't even need a spiralizer. Just heat the oven to 400 degrees, cut a squash in half, roast it flat side down for 20-25 minutes, cool, and string with a fork.

D.I.E.T. #30

Use a food spiralizer to try a new veggie shape, or roast a spaghetti squash and use instead of starchy pasta.

January 31

If you are in a good exercise routine, consider making it more worthwhile by adding an appropriate post workout snack. If you aren't exercising regularly, add something today, and follow it with some post workout fuel. Here's what to eat:

For every hour of exercise, most people need about thirty grams of carb and ten to fifteen grams of protein. Consider that a cup of milk has eight grams of protein and twelve grams of carbohydrate. Make it eight ounces of *chocolate* milk and you will get the same protein, and about thirty grams of carb. For a non-dairy option, try one cup of edamame pods and a choice of fruit for twenty-five grams of carb and ten grams of protein. Or, find a ready to drink shake that meets your needs.

D.I.E.T. #31

Post-fuel your workout. Within 30 minutes of finishing, eat carbs and protein, in about a 2:1 ratio. Notice how afternoon cravings for sweet and salt snacks disappear!

February 1

Portion control is a challenge, especially with delicious food. Somehow, eating bottomless broccoli isn't as appealing as unlimited breadsticks or all you can eat pancakes. It can seem like a measure of will to leave delicious food on your plate.

It could also be a matter of feeling wasteful. But let's consider the damage done to your body from years of cleaning plates. It is okay to leave a little of the good stuff for the dog, or dump it down the drain. Regardless of whether you are out to eat, taking food from home, or eating at home, leave a little starch. If you don't have starch included, leave a little of your favorite part. A sense of control can be found in the ability to do this a few times in a row.

D.I.E.T. #32

Leave a little something on your plate today. Notice and remember how this makes you feel. You can enjoy a new sense of willpower!

February 2

It's Groundhog Day, so why not repeat some success? When you find something that works, it is sensible to keep doing it. The point of D.I.E.T.S. 365 is to accumulate good habits, and to continue the ones that help you reach your goals.

Even though it might only be your second month, you have likely seen that it doesn't matter if you go in order. The point is to go in the right direction, which is toward success. Repeating something over and over will help it to become a habit, which then becomes a lifestyle. Lifestyles work for the long run to improve quantity and quality of life. So flip through the book again, and whether it is eating or training focused, choose an inspiration that will make a big impact on today.

D.I.E.T. #33

Repeat any D.I.E.T. Choose one that allowed you to notice something you didn't notice before, or a strategy you hadn't tried before. If the groundhog saw his shadow today, you may want to have a warm drink while you decide what to repeat!

February 3

If you feel the symptoms of seasonal affective disorder, you are one of as many as 20% of people in the United States alone. "SAD" is a form of major depressive disorder, and affects people in northern climates more often than in sunnier locations. Lack of direct sunlight is also often the cause.

Vitamin D is a fat-soluble vitamin that has been associated with mental health, but also weight control, sleep patterns, and disease risk. Sunlight is the best source, but to get enough direct sunlight every day may not be realistic, so many people take Vitamin D supplements. There are a few rich dietary sources of Vitamin D that can help boost your intake. Three ounces of salmon provides 100% of the RDA for Vitamin D, while 3 ounces of tuna provides around 40%. One cup of fortified milk offers 30%, fortified yogurt comes in at 20%, and an egg yolk gives you 10%.

D.I.E.T. #34

Consider asking your doctor about your Vitamin D status, and consume a rich dietary source today.

February 4

Snacking isn't always bad, especially when choosing a nutrient rich food that provides energy. Foods rich in protein, healthy fats, and fiber can be the best at providing satiety until the next meal, and are also easier to consume in moderation. Eating out of a bowl or on a plate can help too.

Measure or weigh your snack, and take care in coming up with something balanced. It should have *at least* one gram of protein or healthy fats to every three grams of carbohydrate. Try a source of dairy with a carbohydrate, such as cheese and whole grain crackers. Or, go for a serving of nuts and berries. Another way to do it is to pick a food that is already naturally balanced. An easy example is popcorn. One serving of light popcorn includes fifteen grams of carbohydrate, ten grams of fat, and two grams of protein. It also offers three grams of filling fiber and is typically gluten free.

D.I.E.T. #35

Eat popcorn, or another naturally balanced snack. Use an air popper and avoid topping with butter for a lower fat version.

February 5

Pushups are one of the best exercises to get the entire body working. The traditional style can be intimidating if you don't regularly practice them, but you can get your whole body working with a number of variations of pushups. They work the chest, shoulders, back, biceps, triceps, abdominals, and even the legs, all at once.

If you've never attempted them, try pushups with your hands on a wall or the edge of a counter first. Then, move to a version on your knees, or in full push up position on the floor. The rules: have your hands at least shoulder width apart at shoulder height, keep your hips in a line with your heels and the back of your head, and pull the belly muscles in to support the spine. Lower your upper body by bending at the elbows until the chest is near the wall, countertop or floor, keep your legs straight and firm. Exhale and straighten your arms.

D.I.E.T. #36

Do three sets of pushups. Be honest with yourself and do as many as you can with good form. Then stop, rest, and repeat, or do your sets at separate times.

February 6

At the end of a busy day, it's hard to think about what to make for dinner, and the time it will take in preparation and clean up.

Making meals ahead takes time too, but spending the time when you have it is better than when you are tired and stressed. Plan ahead and prepare some ingredients for your slow cooker. It's simple, and it can all be frozen together ahead of time. For example, place rinsed and dried raw chicken breast in a zip top freezer bag along with salsa, canned corn, black beans, and fire roasted tomatoes. Freeze flat and defrost in the fridge the night before you want to cook it. There are many meals that will work in this same prepared-ahead way.

D.I.E.T. #37

Get out the slow cooker! Use fresh ingredients for soup or chili tonight. Or put it on the counter for dinner tomorrow. Remove a meal you have frozen ahead of time, and place in the refrigerator. Once defrosted, place contents in the slow cooker. Set to low for four to eight hours, and enjoy the benefits of planning ahead!

February 7

What is something you can't do? There are certainly things you truly can't do, but there are also things that you are not aware you are capable of. Those are opportunities that are missed due to low confidence or motivation. When you change your mind about it, and become curious if you CAN, that is when positive change is made. Curiosity leads to trial. Then, you realize you are capable of more!

To start that curiosity, think about one thing you did in your past, but "can't" do now? Or something you want to do, but can't imagine it? Do you have a goal that is simple, but not a priority? The word "can't" gets in the way of the word "will." Change those words around today.

D.I.E.T. #38

Pick something you think you can't do. Push yourself and do it today. It could be five more minutes on the treadmill, five more pushups, or it might be cooking dinner at home. Is it eating a vegetable? Change your mind, just for today, and see where it leads you!

February 8

There are many ways to slow down eating. Why slow down? When you chew slower, you allow more sensation in the mouth, which gives you a better awareness of taste. In this way, slowing down can result it better satiety. Physically, it also takes a while to recognize fullness. If you are eating quickly, you may not feel full until you have already overeaten.

Slowing down allows more time for the brain to catch up with the stomach. If food intake is slower, the brain will recognize signals sooner, and the urge to eat will be lessened before you overeat. How do you slow down? One great tip is to enjoy a frozen snack. I like to suggest fruit such as cherries, blueberries, grapes, or sliced bananas. They can be enjoyed straight from the freezer, or thawed a bit. Eat them over yogurt for added protein, or sprinkle them with chia seeds as they thaw for a healthy fat crunch.

D.I.E.T. #39

Freeze a snack. Eating something frozen forces slower consumption, and offers more enjoyment from smaller portions.

February 9

Curbing a sweet tooth is a tough process. Consuming more sugar causes more sugar cravings. Quitting anything cold turkey isn't easy, but with sugar, it is easier than allowing it in moderation. It is a great strategy to attempt avoidance at least once in a while, so try it today. It might help to vocalize your goal to someone you trust. Stick to it, just for twenty-four hours, and you will see your willpower improve!

Added sugar has many names, so be aware that an ingredient label may read: brown sugar, corn sweetener, corn syrup, dextrose, fructose, fruit juice concentrates, glucose, high-fructose corn syrup, honey, invert sugar, lactose, maltose, malt, molasses, raw sugar, sucrose, sugar, or syrup. Avoid foods containing these ingredients.

D.I.E.T. #40

Avoid added sugar today. Added sugar is found in packaged goods, and obviously in the sugar bowl. Make sure you read every label for sugar today, or avoid foods and beverages that have labels. Feel free to consume fruit or dairy, as they are not considered added sugar.

February 10

The way a person practices yoga should be in his or her own style. If directed by a good teacher, the experience can be enhanced, but if yoga is practiced based solely on what an instructor says, it is not truly "yoga." So, do yoga your own way, and while they can be great, don't insist on needing an instructor or a class.

Yoga doesn't directly cause weight loss, but it helps a person lose weight by allowing reduction of stress hormones and by enhancing a person's ability to be in the present moment. This reduces emotional eating and helps in gauging actual physical hunger. Even a few minutes of yoga practice, when performed daily, can improve your ability to make more mindful decisions.

D.I.E.T. #41

Do yoga today. Remember, this means anything from breathing on purpose, to performing "asana" or yoga poses. To be successful you have to avoid judgment, so if you start to criticize yourself, hit the reset button. Keep wiping your mind clear of any criticism for the duration of your practice.

February 11

Eating a better variety of foods will provide you with a better variety of nutrients. Vegetarian or vegan foods can be a way to mix up your entrees and be a little adventurous. Eating at least one meatless meal each week will give your body a break from processing animal proteins, and will perhaps increase your fiber, vitamin, and mineral intake.

Examples of proteins you might use as the focus of your entrée include lentils, tofu, tempeh, edamame, and eggs (if you are going ovo-vegetarian). Including whole grains such as quinoa, chia seeds, and whole wheat pastas can up your protein compared to refined starches, and will offer additional fiber.

D.I.E.T. #42

Make a meatless meal. I like to suggest something somewhat familiar, such as using edamame pasta with a lightened Alfredo sauce, or trying an entrée salad with quinoa and feta cheese on top.
As you feel more adventurous, try more daring ingredients!

February 12

What you see on a plate can definitely affect your appetite. A large plate with appropriate servings of protein, veggies, and starch will appear much different than if you put those servings on a smaller plate. If you are eating from a pan or other serving dish, you are also much more likely to eat a larger portion.

For this reason, it is suggested that meals be served on dessert or salad plates, no larger than nine inches in diameter. In fact, in Europe the average plate already measures that, while in the U.S. many plates are at 12" or more in diameter. Try using smaller plates. When you do, you will likely see a bigger portion and feel more satisfied from a smaller one!

D.I.E.T. #43

Eat from a smaller plate. Choose an appetizer plate for breakfast, a dessert plate for lunch, and a salad plate for dinner. These can range from four to nine inches, but the idea is to fill a smaller plate and stay away from second helpings!

February 13

When you think about exercising with a friend instead of getting on a treadmill in a damp basement, you might not be so depressed about it. Distracting yourself from the work you are doing is helpful, and the time goes by much faster when you have someone to talk to. Including another person also helps you keep your promise to exercise.

If it isn't nice enough to get outside and meet a neighbor, try a local gym or other class studio. Many of these offer a free first class so you can trial the workout. You could also purchase a workout video or follow a youtube session for free. Do it with a friend, spouse, or other family member, in the comfort of one of your home.

D.I.E.T. #44

Get active with a buddy. It will keep you accountable, and offer some fun and socialization. Healthy (not misery) loves company!

February 14

There are lots of foods that are good for your heart, but instead of choosing that Valentine's Day theme, choose to eat a food that you love. It could be healthy, less healthy, or a better version of a less healthy food. What you choose depends on what you want for today.

Healthy foods give you lots of nutrients to feel good about, but less healthy foods also have things to offer such as gratification, and satisfaction. Deprivation is not a maintainable state, so indulging a bit on a holiday can absolutely be appropriate. You can also consider a healthier version of something you love, such as homemade pizza versus greasy takeout varieties. The most important thing is that you value what you are eating and you value the company you are with.

D.I.E.T. #45

Have something you love today, in honor of Valentine's Day! Share it with a significant other, child, or friend. Enjoy the food and the time you get to spend with each other.

February 15

Oatmeal is often thought of as a heart healthy food. Because it is a whole grain, oatmeal contains fiber, and it includes a significant amount of soluble fiber, which has been shown to reduce both cholesterol and blood sugar. A half-cup serving provides four grams of fiber, three of which are soluble.

Fiber is good for your heart and blood sugar, but oats are filling too! Due to the soluble beta-glucan fiber, which dissolves in water, oats increase the feeling of fullness. Adding a bit of protein by cooking it with milk or adding a teaspoon of protein powder can enhance its staying power.

Naturally low in sugar and sodium, oats also contain many vitamins and mineral helpful in energy production. To flavor plain varieties, consider adding smashed berries, vanilla extract, cocoa, peanut butter, or nuts.

D.I.E.T. #46

Eat oatmeal today. It doesn't have to be at breakfast. Oats are a great mid day snack, or any time a hungry tummy needs filling up.

February 16

A clear mind is helpful in improving your decisions. When distracted, it is much easier to make a quick, impulsive choice. Focus on what you are doing in the moment, and consider the risk/benefit of your decision and you will be more likely to choose healthy! How do you get to the clear state of mind?

There are many ways to gain clarity when you are feeling an urge or having a craving. One of the easiest and quickest strategies is to get a breath of fresh air. Even if the weather isn't ideal, taking a quick step outside or opening a window briefly is a great way to reset your mind. You will be taking a healthier action and placing a moment between your urge and your choice.

D.I.E.T. #47

Get some fresh air! Step out on your front or back porch, take a deep breath, and exhale. Stay outside if it's nice, or head back in. Either way, you've made a healthy move today.

February 17

Whole grains can mean anything from whole wheat, oats, corn, or quinoa. Many nutrients are removed when a grain is refined to the white, or processed version. Eat the "whole" thing and you will reap the benefits of additional fiber, protein, vitamins and minerals such as magnesium. Whole grain is more filling, and provides the body with the ingredients for better energy production.

To find whole grains, look for "whole" on the ingredient label, or look for the color brown, when it comes to rice. Be aware that brown doesn't always mean whole grain. It's easy to be tricked with vegetable based foods as well. For example, veggie pastas may or may not contain whole grain, and may include vegetables in powdered or dry forms, which don't provide the natural fibers and absorbable nutrients that whole forms do.

D.I.E.T. #48

Eat only whole grains when you consume starchy foods today. This could be a half-cup serving of oats for breakfast, quinoa for lunch, and brown rice with your dinner.

February 18

Foods recommended for heart health have other benefits too. For example, salmon is full of fats that are healthy for the heart, but also contain protein, and minerals such as calcium. It is efficient to find foods that provide a multitude of benefits, and even if you don't have a condition such as heart disease, it is wise to consume these multifunctional foods daily! Another food with multiple benefits is ground flax seed.

Flax seed is found in whole and ground forms. Whole, it can be used as a topper and in baking, but travels through the body virtually unchanged, providing fiber as a benefit to the digestive tract. When eaten in its ground form it also provides fiber, but offers absorption of its omega three fats, which work to provide the body with anti-inflammatory properties.

D.I.E.T. #49

Include ground flax seed today. Sprinkle over cereal, mix into a smoothie, add to entrees such as meatloaf or soups, or stir into salad dressings. Start with a teaspoon or two per day and advance to a tablespoon at a time.

February 19

Since it's the birthday of my first child, I find today a great day to think like a kid. Reflect on childhood and think back to how you thought about food, if you did. Did food matter that much? Would you rather have played outside or come in for dinner? Did you ask for seconds if you weren't hungry?

Most children see food as necessary when they are hungry, and tend to avoid it when they are not. They understand the feeling of hunger and want to satisfy it. When they have enough, they argue the right to leave food on their plate. While it may be the vegetables they leave, children also tend to eat small portions of everything, so they can get back to what they were doing before the meal.

D.I.E.T. #50

In honor of my first child, eat like a kid today. Think back to how you thought about food, or didn't. Pay attention to things other than second helpings, and be eager to go back to something after your meal.

February 20

Cooking is either something you like or you don't. I don't know anyone who "sort of" likes to cook. Maybe it's the cleaning up part, or the feeling that it is hard to please everyone, or maybe it is lack of creativity or energy. Getting something new into the kitchen is sometimes helpful to sparking an old, or a new, love for cooking.

My favorite things to freshen up the kitchen include spatulas that flip, stir, and scrape, fresh cutting boards, or a new serving dish. A footed dessert bowl works great for serving berries at the table, and a whimsical spoon may get your kids to eat their veggies. It can be as simple as that, or can be more complicated such as a new slow cooker or fancy blender.

D.I.E.T. #51

Buy a new kitchen gadget. You don't have to spend a lot of money or go to an upscale cooking store, but choose something that will inspire you to try a new food or a different way of eating.

February 21

Sometimes we complicate our lives unintentionally, such as when too many things are added to the calendar or when we communicate the wrong message to someone important. Eating should be simplified, because when there are too many things to think about, giving up is imminent.

A simple way to eat less has nothing to do with what you are eating, but instead, how. Put your main utensil in your non-dominant hand, and slower eating is now imminent! You may have heard this tactic before because it works, unless you are ambidextrous. You will fill up faster on a smaller volume of food.

D.I.E.T. #52

Put your eating utensil in your non-dominant hand. Do this at every meal today, and notice how it makes you more mindful of each poke of the fork or scoop of the spoon. You may want to try this in private or with people who know what you are doing, in case you make a mess!

February 22

For a long time, eating fat was taboo. It was seen as unhealthy for your heart and weight, and low fat versions of most everything were made available. We now know that fats have an essential role in creating long lasting energy and satiety, are healthy for your heart, and can actually help you become leaner.

To eat more fat in a healthy way, start out with plant-based fats by consuming more nuts and seeds. Add ground flaxseed or avocados to smoothies and include marine based omega three fats from fish. Changing your oil of choice to olive is perhaps the simplest habit to swap. If the taste is hard to get used to, try a light version for a milder flavor, but also note that these refined versions have less of the beneficial properties compared to extra virgin olive oil.

D.I.E.T. #53

Trade all of the oil you use today for olive oil. Place it in a bottle near where you cook, prepare a salad dressing with olive oil as the base, and use it anytime you would use butter or margarine. A drizzle of olive oil is delicious over veggies.

February 23

There are many reasons to exercise early in the day, but getting some activity toward the end of the day can be helpful too. Doing something after dinner helps digestion, relieves stress, and decreases the likelihood of eating dessert, or a bedtime snack.

Something as simple as getting into a routine of walking around the block post-meal can help to replace other less healthy options, such as plopping on the couch, having a drink, or eating sugary snacks. Walking briskly will burn a few calories, but the main reason for this walk is to avoid other habits and improve the body's use of the dinner meal.

D.I.E.T. #54

Take a walk after dinner. It doesn't have to be outside, but if the weather permits, the outdoors can be refreshing. If you must do your activity inside, consider an exercise machine or just a walk around the house, outside of the kitchen. Doing this daily can reap great results!

February 24

There are many ways to enjoy vegetables, but perhaps one of the easiest and most likeable ways to prepare them is by steaming. Contrary to some sources, steaming veggies does not reduce their nutritional value enough to negate the benefits. Fiber and nutrients are preserved when steaming vegetables versus boiling them. Additionally, steamed vegetables might be consumed in greater quantities, due to the ease of eating soft foods versus raw.

Steaming can be done with a simple pot of water and steam basket. Make sure the water is below the level of the steam basket, and boil just long enough for the vegetables to soften. Steaming can also be done in the microwave, without water, using a steam bag or other specialized container.

D.I.E.T. #55

Steam some veggies today! Make them in a big batch if you like leftovers. It's easy to add a vinaigrette dressing and store them in the fridge for snacking. You can also store them as is and pack them in your lunch.

February 25

Spacing meals out is a great way to help your body rest and reset. Hormones like insulin rise when eating, so that blood sugar can be normalized. Continue to eat and insulin continues to be secreted. Alternately, give your body a break and insulin levels will normalize. Many people make the mistake of "grazing," and eating all day long. Especially if a person is eating the wrong foods, this habit can wreak havoc!

If you have diabetes, this may be common knowledge, but everyone can benefit from the idea of eating regularly spaced meals with carbs, proteins, and healthy fats. What does regularly spaced mean? Typically, you should leave three or four hours between eating times, but athletes or very active people might eat more often.

D.I.E.T. #56

Wait three hours or more between meals and/or snacks. Notice if your body gets hungry, or if you reach for food before the time is up. This is a great exercise for improving awareness!

February 26

A simple way to be more efficient with eating healthy is to use recipes that allow for doubling. Leftovers are then utilized for lunches, or for preparing a quick dinner. Meal "prep" can be interpreted in many ways, but the process of making a double recipe is simple and quite effective!

Choose a family favorite, to be certain it is one you want to double! Casserole style meals work well for this. Some of my favorites include Tex-Mex style lasagna made by layering corn tortillas, lean ground meat, seasonings, black beans, corn or other veggies, and cheese. Use a freezable container for the second dish and write the date and contents on the outside. Don't forget about it!

D.I.E.T. #57

Make two meals at once! Freeze the uneaten portion, typically after cooking it thoroughly. To reheat, thaw in the refrigerator and heat in the oven until bubbly, usually twenty to thirty minutes.

February 27

Pick action. If you have a hard time starting something you may need to stop thinking about it, and just take the first step. Some people find that leaving a gym bag in the car helps them steer toward the gym. Others leave their shoes sitting untied by the garage door.

It's easy to fall into a pattern of feeling like everything is too hard to do. So forget about doing everything, and pick one thing. Then release the thought that you should be, or could be, doing something else with your time. Just put one foot in front of the other.

D.I.E.T. #58

Commit to one ACTION. Whatever it is you are working on, take a step toward it. Don't give yourself any option except to lace up your shoes and get started, or head to the grocery store for dinner ingredients. Make the first move, and the next move will follow.

February 28

Eating foods on purpose is a great habit to be in. Avoiding certain foods can be depressing and defeating, so it is often more beneficial to focus on certain things to *include*. Nuts are a great source of heart healthy fats, fiber, and a bit of protein. Certain nuts are better in these categories than others. Walnuts are one of my favorites because of the omega 3 fats they contain, which are shown to reduce cholesterol, and their calorie density can improve satiety.

Having a goal of eating a single serving of walnuts today is specific (S), measurable (M), action-oriented (A), realistic (R), and time sensitive (T). It is not only S.M.A.R.T, it is beneficial to your health in many ways. Try adding them to oatmeal or a smoothie, or atop salad, if you don't love the taste of them plain. Use a measured one-ounce portion, or about ¼ cup of walnuts.

D.I.E.T. #59

Eat walnuts today to improve your health. Notice if they affect your appetite, or if you feel energized for longer.

February 29

Leap year only comes around every four years, so if you are reading this consider yourself lucky! Goals that may come to mind today could be skipping breakfast or skipping exercise, but let's be healthier since this is a rare occasion! Consider setting some long-term goals.

I usually like to suggest mini short-term goals, or daily goals. A close second is setting short-term goals that help you achieve your long-term vision. Accumulating goals paves a road to success. Reviewing your vision for the long-term future is appropriate on this once-every-four years-holiday.

D.I.E.T. #60

Record 4 goals you want to accomplish before the next Leap Year. Remember, you have 1,460 days, so aim high. If it's a weight loss goal, make it challenging but realistic for the long term. Other goals, such as achieving normal cholesterol values, improving other disease states, or better lab results is also very helpful and appropriate for the long run.

March 1

A new gadget or utensil is fun and can be motivating, but a new drinking container is specific to improving one thing--hydration. Focusing on improving hydration will secretly help you achieve better results in your other health goals. You might have a cupboard full of water bottles. That's great, you might not have to spend any money!

Get out an old one, or cave and buy something new. It is important that you have something you can take with you to refill throughout the day. There are many brands of fancy, expensive cups and thermal ware, but you don't have to spend a lot of money if you don't want to. Choose a BPA free item. Consider whether a straw or wide mouth will help you drink more.

D.I.E.T. #61

Find an old favorite drinking vessel, or buy a new one. It could be a water bottle, cup, or thermal mug. Consider adding ice, a straw, and/or fresh fruit to flavor water on the run. In any case, take your water with you. If it's accessible, you are more likely to drink it.

March 2

Omega 3 fats are a type of polyunsaturated fats, and are capable of lowering cholesterol, specifically triglycerides. They are also considered anti-inflammatory, which makes them helpful in overall body function. The marine omega 3 fats DHA and EPA are most plentiful in fish such as salmon, but are also found in popular fish such as sea bass, trout, mackerel, oysters, herring and sardines.

It is recommended to consume about 8 ounces per week of a variety of seafood, or to obtain about 250 mg per day EPA and DHA combined. Three ounces of wild or farmed salmon contains about 1500 mg while three ounces of trout offers over 800 and canned tuna provides about 200 mg. This is data from the U.S. Department of Agriculture, Agricultural Research Service, Nutrient Data Laboratory, 2015.

D.I.E.T. #62

Eat fish today! It doesn't have to be the powerhouse salmon, and a small portion at one meal will do. Fish offers omega 3 and also a lean source of protein to satisfy you until your next meal or snack.

March 3

Go where temptations are plenty, and you are sure to give in. Whether you are at work, or at home, or working from home, access to tempting food is everything. Take yourself away from the temptation, and the urge can be minimized and easier to manage. Avoiding the kitchen as much as possible keeps you from thinking about food all day long.

Of course you need to eat, fill up your glass of water, and possibly make an after school snack for the kids. I'm talking about the between meal times. At work, stay out of the break room and take a walk outside instead. At home, head to the laundry room and fold clothes, or better yet, head to that long list of errands you are behind on!

D.I.E.T. #63

Stay out of the kitchen today, except to prepare and eat meals. If you are distracted, or think about what is around to eat, you are surely to eat when you aren't physically hungry.

March 4

On March 4, 1993, Jim Valvano was dying of cancer and gave an amazing speech at the first ever ESPY awards. In his speech, Valvano said it was a full day if you can laugh, think, and cry. It's true that feeling emotions is important to your short and long term health. Keeping things bottled up creates stress and unhappiness, and causes the body additional harm.

It might take reading funny memes to make you laugh, or watching a movie to be tearful, but emotions are healthy. If you can be in a moment of sadness or loneliness and cry through it, it is a great release. Laughing can also bring you to tears so let loose and let it out! The sensation of feeling is an important part of your journey.

D.I.E.T. #64

Move your emotions today. Feel free to having feelings, and don't try to numb yourself. Instead, sit with feelings, and let them pass with tears, laughter, or deep thought.

March 5

Is there such a thing as a super food? There are lots of foods that have benefits and are ultra healthy. By my definition, "super" means a food has multiple functions or benefits to the body. These might include a food's ability to improve cholesterol, blood sugar, or blood pressure numbers, improve bowel, brain, or muscular function, or possibly reduce risk for chronic disease.

You will have to include more than just one serving of one super food to see a difference, but consider eating super foods more often, with variety. Some of the foods on my super-foods list that are readily available include: olive oil, blueberries, avocados, pomegranate seeds, salmon, chia seeds, ground flax seeds, and oats.

D.I.E.T. #65

Include a super-food today. Don't worry if you can't find acai berries or goji berries. Top oatmeal with ground flax seed and blueberries and you'll have three in one meal!

March 6

Setting the atmosphere is a big deal when it comes to success at mealtimes. Create a relaxing place to eat, instead of having chaos set the tone. This can be challenging with kids, or with a busy schedule. Taking time to slow down and enjoy eating requires intention and practice!

Making the eating environment relaxing usually has to be a priority, so try making it one and see how it affects your portion control, satisfaction, and need for dessert! Lighting a candle is a great way to set the mood and purposefully show your devotion to relaxing through a meal. When you need to put your fork down or drink some water, look at the candle to remind you to relax and enjoy!

D.I.E.T. #66

Light a candle today. Put it on the table and look at it for a little reminder to relax, especially if you have had a challenging day.

March 7

Spending lots of money on dieting, only to gain the weight back is frustrating. Typically, more money spent does not equal long-term success. Getting inspired on a daily basis can be hard, and it might feel like you need to spend money on fancy supplements, diet plans and workout clothes. However, a simple, small purchase might do the same thing for your motivation.

Purchase something you can use to your benefit for years down the road. You might not think of a cooking magazine to fit into this category, but if you find a few recipes that you enjoy, it can change more than just today. After you've tried them, cut out recipes you like, and create a file of meals you will make again.

D.I.E.T. #67

Buy a cooking magazine. Browse through them before you select one, to make sure the recipes include realistic ingredients that you like. Even if you don't like cooking, creating something you can enjoy at home is empowering.

March 8

I know there are other people out there like me who crave the morning time, for their cup of coffee and a bit of peace and quiet. Even if you don't like coffee, you probably have a routine that you stick to in the morning hours. It is typical and common for this to be the "easy" time of day.

Caffeine might offer an initial energy boost, but it is possible to extend the period of time in the morning when you have that increased productivity. Adding one half to one tablespoon of useful fats to your morning coffee can help extend the effect of caffeine, and can help your body begin to break down fats for energy. I suggest a medium chain triglyceride source (or MCT), including MCT oil, or coconut oil. If you absolutely won't drink coffee, add this to a homemade smoothie instead. Notice how your energy is extended and the afternoon is a bit easier.

March 9

Needing something else after a meal is a common concern for many people. It is often described as a need for something sweet. Sometimes a person continues to eat, snacking into the next meal without really taking a break. This can be very hard to overcome, especially if it's a habit to give into the urge.

Having something healthy and refreshing is one solution. For example, a bowl of fresh berries in the fridge can stave off the sweet tooth. For many, the desire for stronger sweet satisfaction drives them to chocolate, or a more dense dessert such as ice cream. While I don't like to recommend restricting or avoiding, many times the taste left in the mouth after a meal drives an urge, and brushing your teeth can solve this problem.

D.I.E.T. #69

Brush your teeth after every meal/snack today. Take a travel toothbrush with you, or keep a travel mouthwash in your pocket. If you forget your toothbrush or don't have the courage to brush in public, swishing mouthwash can also do the trick.

March 10

Having company in the kitchen can make the experience more enjoyable, especially if you give your help specific tasks in the preparation of your meal. If you don't have kids, enlist your spouse, roommate, or a friend to do the chopping, stirring, measuring, or dishes.

Show your kitchen guest the recipe you are following, then delegate the in between tasks that help the meal come together. A helper can prepare a side dish while you put the main course together, or can gather condiments, drinks, and silverware. It may depend on what you are cooking, but there are many tasks that can be time consuming and may have to be done at the same time you are doing something else.

D.I.E.T. #70

Enlist a helper in the kitchen such as a child, spouse, or friend. I've heard that too many cooks in the kitchen can be a problem, but designating space for chopping, mixing, and garnishing is easy and can make the meal come together quickly, and with less anxiety!

March 11

Balancing the gut bacteria is a daily challenge for many people who suffer from IBS or other digestive conditions. Diagnosing a gastrointestinal problem can be a difficult guessing game too, and is usually based on symptoms. If you have food sensitivities, are trying to lose weight, or have other chronic diseases, balancing the good bacteria in your gut can be a step towards relieving your symptoms. Even if you don't have stomach issues, adding a probiotic or prebiotic-containing food is great for overall health!

Eating a food versus taking a pill can be a more conservative and overall helpful approach. Some of the more common foods to try: yogurt (even as little as one to two tablespoons), artichokes, or one of the three "k's:" kefir, kimchi, or kombucha.

D.I.E.T. #71

Eat a probiotic or prebiotic food. Hippocrates said, "all health begins in the gut," so make sure you already have, or are working toward creating a healthy gut environment.

March 12

Starting at the beginning, or using a "baseline" measurement can be depressing, or it can be motivating. It depends on how you look at it. Using a scale to measure your progress is positive. Using it to condemn yourself, or self-sabotage is obviously not. Keep a scale out of sight, and pull it out once a week or less, preferably on the same day, to determine how your habits are affecting your weight.

Look at it as an experiment, instead of an emotional experience. Write down your weight in a logbook and put the book away until the next week. Consider that traveling, weight training, heavy endurance training, menstrual cycles and other hormones can greatly affect your numbers.

D.I.E.T. #72

Weigh yourself and record your result, then put the scale away for a week. Don't consider it a trend until you see three to four weeks of weight change, upward or down.

March 13

Snacking on vegetables might sound cliché and unreasonable for some, but this habit is a really great one that is easy to get used to, even if you don't like many veggies. The crunch of something fresh and hydrating can provide enough satisfaction to get you through to the next meal. The trick is to have it ready, clean and in plain sight.

My favorites to clean and snack on are some of the more simple choices, but feel free to get fancy. Try baby bok choy instead of organic spinach leaves. Broccoli slaw is easy to eat a handful of, as are baby carrots and celery. Sliced cucumbers, bell peppers, and mushrooms might be my favorites to eat straight out of the fridge.

D.I.E.T. #73

Eat like a bunny. Since it's his birthday and spring is near, this is dedicated to my father in law for his healthy habits of eating lettuce by the leaf, and carrots by the handful.

March 14

There's something about verbalizing your goals that sets them alive. Committing yourself is important, and telling someone else about your goal is an important part of the step. It could be through a Facebook page or a special social media group, but telling it in person is also very beneficial. You may be able to enlist a coworker or friend to help you stay accountable!

Decide on something specific and tell someone you trust. It could be just one person, or if you like more group accountability, announce it more dramatically! Remember to share your long-term goal, and a short-term goal or plan for achieving it. You don't have to give all of the background reasons, but let people know that you are looking forward to sharing your progress.

D.I.E.T. #74

Publicize a goal. When you share a goal, it is much harder to stray from your path.

March 15

It's hard to be creative at the end of a long day. If you can manage to come up with an easy recipe to cook with items you already have on hand, it is your lucky day! If not, go to the computer for advice. Search any basic meal item you have in the house and you are bound to find thousands of recipes. Better yet, get more specific and type in a few ingredients.

Some of my favorite, most common searches include chicken and broccoli, salmon with rice, and healthy pasta entrees. This results in thousands of recipes, so you may want to add the descriptors of "healthy," "lightened," or "low carb."

D.I.E.T. #75

Search the Internet for a recipe, using a specific ingredient or ingredients you have on hand. Choose a recipe then move any necessary ingredients from the freezer to the fridge, to defrost throughout the day.

March 16

Finding a fun activity to incorporate into the day is a great way to stay active and not have to try too hard. Choose something portable, or do exercise that only requires your body, then commit a few times today to devote to your activity.

A portable piece of equipment that can remind you of childhood is a jump rope. You don't have to spend much, and you don't have to do it long to notice an increased heart rate and a bit of breathlessness. If you don't want to do high impact jumping, consider skipping one leg to the other, or simple swinging the rope around and stepping one foot over at a time.

D.I.E.T. #76

Jump rope. I suggest three bouts of this mini workout. Complete 3 one-minute rounds with rest in between, or advance to longer sets with rest in between. Then, repeat this two to three times today.

March 17

I'm not Irish, but I know the importance of this holiday to the culture of the Irish! In honor of them, in addition to wearing green, I always like to cook something green. While corn beef and cabbage may be the tradition, you can also make something colorful as a side dish or as the main entrée for dinner.

I suggest green entrée items such as edamame pasta with olive oil and parmesan, basil pesto as a base for homemade pizza or pasta dishes, and spinach salads. You can do side dishes such as roasted broccoli or peas. You can also make green smoothies full of kale, avocado, Greek yogurt, and milk or juice of your choice.

D.I.E.T. #77

Cook something green today, or be adventurous and try a green smoothie! Just because it's St. Patrick's Day doesn't mean you have to overindulge. Don't just celebrate by having a stout beer.

March 18

Getting your digestive tract to cooperate with your body can be a challenge. Sometimes eating healthy can cause MORE symptoms, such as gas, bloating, and bowel irregularities. Going slow when making changes can help ease some of the possible "shock to your system."

Research suggests that drinking vinegar prior to your largest meal can help digestion and help lower blood sugar responses to meals. To see if it works for you, go slow. Dilute one tablespoon of apple cider vinegar in two tablespoons water. Drink it right before your largest meal. If it doesn't make you feel one way or the other, it's okay. This is a harmless habit to trial for a bit of time, to see if it in fact helps your digestive tract.

D.I.E.T. #78

Drink vinegar. Try it today, and continue if you like the results. Vinegar will assist the breakdown of your meal, and may delay carbohydrate breakdown, which can result in better blood glucose responses.

March 19

Relaxing is important to health for many reasons. Today, experience the effect of breathing on your overall sense of anxiety. This requires only a few moments of quiet, at least a few times today. If you find that it is helpful, do it whenever you become anxious or emotional.

Set your alarm and practice this breath activity at three pre-determined times. If you like, you can insert more times throughout the day. You can perform this in any environment, but a quiet spot is preferable. Close your eyes if possible, or focus your gaze on a certain spot. Breathe in through your nose counting to five in your head slowly. Then, exhale through your nose, counting to five slowly. Repeat this three to five times.

D.I.E.T. #79

Practice breathing today. Try to think of nothing at all while you are breathing. Just count. If your eyes are closed, imagine the numbers going across a black screen.

March 20

Choosing to eat only fresh foods might sound simple, and it is. I won't say it's easy though! This diet includes the complete avoidance of packaged foods including bread, pasta, and cereal, and anything else in the inner aisles of the grocery store. In addition, drink only liquids without labels. Water, tea, and coffee (if brewed at home, not purchased in a bottle) are considered fresh for today.

Packaged produce such as lettuce mixes and cherry tomatoes are allowed, but avoid processed items such as the salads with dressing included and ranch dips, etc. Choose mostly things without wrappers at all. However, dairy is allowed, as is meat and chicken. Just purchase it without added ingredients. Bulk bins where you can buy nuts and seeds also carry grains, which are fine if you cook them yourself.

D.I.E.T. #80

Eat only fresh today. It's the first day of spring. It's also my spring baby's birthday! An easy way to follow this diet is to stay out of the pantry and freezer. It's only for one day!

March 21

Drinking more water is a theme of DIETS 365. But how, you ask? There are lots of ways to increase hydration, and lots of suggestions out there. One tip that works for a variety of reasons is to count your sips.

One large sip, or gulp, is about one ounce of water. To estimate your gulp, measure 4 ounces of water, and see how many normal sized swallows it takes to drink all of it. Then, set a goal to drink sixty-four gulps or more today. (Hint--the trick is to count!) This is easier if you commit to drinking at least 4 gulps every time you have the opportunity. Don't just sip all day on the same glass, but drink it in two "gulpings," then refill it.

D.I.E.T. #81

Count your ounces. You'll more easily keep track of your water intake if you take more than one sip at a time. And, you'll meet your goal more quickly!

March 22

Substituting one ingredient for another can be an easy way to lighten up a recipe, but it is also a great way to boost nutrients in a recipe. One food that gets substituted quite often is an egg. Not only are they easy to run out of, but many people like to eat eggs for breakfast and are trying to limit them in other parts of the day. So, common substitutes include applesauce, Greek yogurt, or canned pumpkin in baking.

Another great substitute that seconds as a nutrient boost is ground flax seed which can be used in baking to mimic an egg. Simply mix one tablespoon of this omega 3 rich fiber source into two tablespoons water. Use it as you would an egg in any recipe. It doesn't work well as an actual egg, if you were wondering, but its properties are similar, without the cholesterol and saturated fat.

D.I.E.T. #82

Use a "flax" egg today. Try it in any recipe that calls for an egg. You can double it too, if your recipe asks for more than one egg.

March 23

Make a plan, even a few hours ahead of time, and you will be much more likely to succeed today. It doesn't have to be elaborate, but if you set the ingredients out, you will almost always come home and cook. If you don't have a plan for dinner, you are more likely to stop and pick something up. In addition to that, if someone else is home first, the suggestion to eat out may be intercepted by the sight of dinner ingredients.

Probably obvious, but leaving the protein course in the fridge is necessary. However, set canned goods and bowls/pans out to create your meal. Place your recipe in plain sight, chop vegetables, and prep anything else you can ahead of time.

D.I.E.T. #83

Put dinner ingredients on the counter, ahead of time. Before you leave in the morning, set yourself up for dinner success. You will save yourself time, money, and the need for willpower!

March 24

While "diet" foods can keep some people from consuming too many calories, they can also be full of ingredients that aren't very natural. Some of these ingredients can cause stomach upset and other gastrointestinal problems. One such ingredient is artificial sweetener.

While not harmful in small quantities, sweeteners can cause a person to crave more sugar, causing them to overeat. They can also disrupt the balance of bacteria in the gut. Most of the time, small amounts don't cause a problem, but pay attention to the amount you consume today. Read labels and avoid anything with aspartame, acesulfame K, sucralose, saccharin, stevia, and sugar alcohols xylitol and sorbitol. There are other artificial sweeteners, but these are the most common.

D.I.E.T. #84

Forgo artificial sweeteners. Notice if you feel any different, and if this is difficult for you. Become more aware of all of the places where sweeteners can hide.

March 25

Helping out around the house can be a great way to add activity. If you are typically in charge, there may be a few things that don't always get done, or that you are not 100% responsible for. Not only can you make someone's day by possibly owning his or her task, but you can add some activity and feel good about it too!

Choose something such as gathering trash from all of the cans around the house, or doing an extra load of laundry. Vacuuming, organizing closets, or cleaning out the garage can be serious calorie burners. These little things will add to your activity, and may keep you away from the kitchen, where you might otherwise be snacking!

D.I.E.T. #85

Add one unusual task for yourself today. While the task itself may not be unusual, pick something you wouldn't ordinarily be doing. Completing an extra "project," will give you a great sense of accomplishment today!

March 26

Everyone needs reminders sometimes. If you find yourself eating mindlessly or sitting still for too long, a reminder might be helpful. A simple item around your wrist can keep you focused on your goal today. I suggest a rubber band, but a hair tie or a bracelet can work too. Choose something you don't normally wear around your wrist.

Now, choose something you need a reminder for. I suggest a rubber band to keep people from eating when they are not hungry, or to remind them to get out of a seated position once or twice per hour. It might be that every time you notice your wrist you take a drink of water.

D.I.E.T. #86

Wear a rubber band around your wrist. Then, decide what you are committing to today. Every time you glance at the item, remind yourself of your goal today. (Hint: Don't wear sleeves that cover the item, or roll them up a bit today!)

March 27

There is something about writing with a pen and paper that can't be replicated on a smart phone or computer. Keeping track of what you eat can be done in a variety of ways. I like using applications that can analyze your intake, but it is also helpful to take a pen to the paper and be committed to recording food intake in a notebook.

If you'd rather be high tech, just try this for today. Write down everything you eat, as you eat it. You may find that it isn't worth grabbing your journal for a handful of candy or a late night snack. It is helpful to keep this food record and reflect on how you can improve your choices. If you want to, plug it into your favorite app tomorrow, have it analyzed, and reflect on how it may have changed your intake.

D.I.E.T. #87

Write down what you eat today. Fancy colored pens or pencil, it doesn't matter! Be aware of how this journaling activity may have affected your choices.

March 28

Counting how many times you chew when you are eating a meal is an exercise in awareness that can help with digestion and overall calorie intake. To slow down eating is often beneficial, especially if you are one who normally eats fast. Take a baseline count. That is, don't change how you normally eat, but count how many times you chew a regularly sized fork or spoonful of food. Then, add ten chews to the next similarly sized bite.

Chewing more increases satisfaction for three main reasons. One, you allow food to reach more taste areas of your tongue and give your tongue more surface area of food to taste. Two, you break food down more before it reaches your stomach. Thirdly, it takes longer when you chew more, so the stomach can recognize fullness sooner.

D.I.E.T. #88

Count your "chews." Then add more to each bite you take. Do this every time you eat today.

March 29

It is helpful to have accountability when trying to develop lifelong habits. Whether you tell your accountability partner about his/her role is up to you. Regardless, today is devoted to recognizing a struggle and leaning on someone for help.

Being aware of your struggle is the first part. It may only be a twinge of a craving that you know you can stave off, but use the opportunity to practice taking an action that will help you remember that you are not alone. Then, when more difficult challenges come along, you will remember to lean on your "person". When you experience a moment of struggle, whether food or stress related, send a text, make a phone call, or use social media. It isn't critical that your support person answer, and it also isn't important that you tell the story of your struggle. Simply reach out to say hello.

D.I.E.T. #89

Use your phone-a-friend. Taking positive action in difficult times can remind you that you aren't alone, and can give you the change in direction you need in the moment.

March 30

Meal prep can be a daunting thought, but it doesn't have to mean prepping full course dinners and gourmet lunches to go. Making something to keep on hand for quick snacking is meal prep at its best! It is simple and most helpful to fix grab and go items that can build a lunch, or offer in between energy at work, school, or other activities.

One of my favorite items to add to the day is a hard-boiled egg. Heavy in protein and minerals, eggs are a great snack to fill up in between meals, and can be paired with fruit, cheese, and nuts to build a balanced lunch. To make them even more convenient, peel a few after they are done, and keep in a sealed container. If you like them pickled, peel, then add to an empty jar of pickle juice or olive brine. They last longer than plain peeled eggs and offer a unique taste!

D.I.E.T. #90

Make hard-boiled eggs. I like to make them a dozen at a time, but consider how many people will eat them, and cook as many as you will consume in about three days.

March 31

March is supposed to go in like a lion and out like a lamb, but it doesn't seem to go that way where I live. No matter what the weather is today, take it easy on yourself. Do some gentle yoga (think, lamb-like!) or commit to bedtime stretching. You could also take a nap or get a relaxing massage. Consider this a "rest" day, and practice some purposeful recovery.

Recovery is rejuvenating to the body and the mind. Today's healthy habit is to take a break from your intense efforts! This doesn't mean eating poorly or being completely sedentary. It means taking time to appreciate yourself and your efforts. Giving your body physical recovery from intense work is important, and giving your mind a break is critical as well.

D.I.E.T. #91

Take a "rest" day and help March go out like a lamb, even if Mother Nature isn't cooperating!

April 1

I'm not one to be overly creative with silly holidays like April Fools, but I also tend to forget about this day, and get tripped up by others who like to celebrate. If it keeps you on your toes today, have a little fun with a meal or two! Make a silly dinner such as meatloaf cake (layer meatloaves with mashed potatoes, using two eight inch round pans) or do meatloaf cupcakes instead. "Frost" with mashed potatoes, and garnish with cherry tomatoes. It really does look like dessert!

Alternately, you can choose to cook breakfast for dinner or have your kids or spouse cook the meal. Now *that's* funny! By all means, don't forget about April Fools, and be on the lookout for others trying to trip you up. Keep up with your progress and remember to stay on the course when temptations (or tricks) come along!

D.I.E.T. #92

Fool someone with a healthy spin on dinner, or at a minimum, stay on your path toward healthy today.

April 2

It can be hard to get enough protein, especially if you are trying to cut back on meat, one of the most dense sources of protein you can eat. Focusing on getting enough can be a great goal, as it is a positive thinking, eye opening process. Having one thing to track, and a goal that is not related to avoiding something can be motivating, and will teach you more about what kinds of calories you are eating.

Aim for at least half a gram per pound of your weight. If you are severely overweight, average your ideal weight with your current weight, use that number and eat half a gram of protein per pound. Look for protein from meat, chicken, poultry, fish, but also eggs, dairy, soy, legumes, and seeds. If needed, supplement with protein powders or bars for a boost to your numbers.

D.I.E.T. #93

Count your protein grams today. Be aware of your normal intake, and what you need to change to meet your goal. For example, swap refined carbohydrate based foods for high quality protein sources.

April 3

Having a plan recorded in plain sight is helpful when trying to make progressive change happen. Putting that plan in your sight, and in the vision of others who live with you can give you a sense of accountability. To make this happen inexpensively, quickly, and effectively, use a board you can write on and erase. I have a chalkboard at home, but it gets messy and I don't love to write with chalk. A white board can be fun, and if you have children, they will love to "decorate" your plan!

Most often, a week at a time is best, but choose to write on your board daily, weekly, or by the month. At the very least, add the dates and your main goals. Record the protein you will have for dinner, if not the daily meal plan, how you will get exercise in, and perhaps a motivational quote or your long-term goal.

D.I.E.T. #94

Use a dry erase board or chalkboard. A mini board might work for daily goals, or select a monthly calendar board for a longer-term plan.

April 4

Unless it triggers migraines or you have another intolerance to it, dark chocolate is a rich, satisfying treat full of benefits. Dark chocolate is a more concentrated form of milk chocolate. It contains more of the nutrient-rich cacao bean than milk chocolate or semi-sweet varieties. As chocolate decreases in percent of cacao, the sugar content increases, and benefits decrease. It, in fact, becomes more "diluted."

An appropriate serving of dark chocolate is one half to one ounce. This equates to between fifteen and thirty grams, if you are measuring it on a scale. This portion might also equate to a "square," when eating it from a bar or package, but weighing it is smart! A serving of dark chocolate can offer a sweet, rich taste when searching for something else to satisfy and mark the end of a meal. It offers the most flavonoids and nutritional benefit, with less sugar than other varieties of chocolate.

D.I.E.T. #95

Eat dark chocolate. It will help you satisfy cravings in a healthier way, and can help you avoid further snacking.

April 5

Distractions happen all day long. Trying to separate eating from other activities is a great way to bring more awareness to your food intake. Not only will you make wiser choices, but you might also be better satisfied with fewer calories and more nutrients. There are many strategies in D.I.E.T.S. 365 to help you be less distracted. Today, remove your computer or laptop from your eating space.

Eating by the computer is wildly popular, due to our need to multitask and be productive. It also causes more interference and mindless eating than any other distraction I've come across. When you eat by the computer, you might forget what you ate, get less enjoyment, and will likely desire additional snacks later in the day.

D.I.E.T. #96

Avoid eating by your computer. Doing so will encourage more chewing and better digestion, and will remind you later in the day that you really don't need that extra snack.

April 6

If you are trying to be less distracted and want to be even more focused, try devoting a few moments prior to eating to practice gratitude. No matter what your religious beliefs, being thankful for food is a critical step toward eating an appropriate amount. If you are grateful and see eating as a privilege, you will eventually eat to nourish your body more often than you will as a glutton or to cope with emotions.

Using prayer or meditation or having a small devotion you repeat before starting to eat will slow you down and remind you to eat for the purpose of nourishing instead of coping or devouring. As a suggestion, use the following: "I am grateful for the opportunity to nourish my body with the food I'm about to eat."

D.I.E.T. #97

Pray or meditate before you eat. You can add more or change the above devotion, but using a simple line prior to eating a meal or snack can be life changing.

April 7

Getting enough protein is so important that is it repeated throughout D.I.E.T.S. 365. There are many solutions as to how to achieve the right protein intake, which is why it is revisited on so many days. By the end of the year, you will have tried many different methods!

Animal products are a simple way to consume protein, but plant proteins show many benefits too. There are many reasons to include soy protein specifically, including its various phytochemicals, bone health, and its ability to lower cholesterol levels. Soy protein is easy to consume in products such as soymilk, cheese and yogurt, along with soybeans in the form of edamame, tempeh, or tofu.

D.I.E.T. #98

Eat soy today. If you've never had it, I suggest starting with edamame or a low sugar flavored soymilk. One serving of protein is 7-8 grams. In volume, this equates to a half-cup serving of edamame or one cup of soymilk.

April 8

With so many activities going on at once, many people rely on phones or computer calendars to stay organized. Work calendars are often synced with personal calendars. While it is helpful to have activities and work recorded in one place, it can be greatly beneficial to plan healthy lifestyles on paper. Leave this in a place where you and others in the household can add and make notes.

Post the calendar or planner in an agreed upon spot, and refer to it daily. For workouts, make sure you add to the calendar on at least a weekly basis. Plan meals by taking a quick inventory of your food options, and plan workouts as priorities around work and family activities. Commit to meals and exercise by writing them down and checking them off.

D.I.E.T. #99

Buy a planner or wall calendar, or dig out the one you bought last December! A planner is a simple and cheap investment to help you achieve your priceless goals.

April 9

As long as you're not allergic, eating nuts is a great way to get more healthy fats, fiber, and protein in your diet. They can provide long lasting energy and satisfaction, but being careful of your serving size is important. Due to their high fat content, nuts are an energy dense food, meaning there are a lot of calories in a small volume.

A serving size of most nuts is one fourth of a cup, or one ounce, but most people agree that a portion like that is hard to stick to. To make it easier, slow down your eating by choosing nuts with a shell. Picking apart peanuts at a ball game or shelling a few pistachios at your desk can offer a healthy distraction, and can keep you from eating handfuls at a time.

D.I.E.T. #100

Eat nuts from a shell today. The simplest are peanuts and pistachios, but you can also find walnuts, brazil nuts, almonds, pecans, and many seeds in shelled forms. Just make sure you have a nutcracker if necessary!

April 10

Moving heavy weights around and sprinting until you puke isn't necessary. It just isn't. Exercise can be simplified by using your body weight. Today, focus on doing something challenging with your body.

Walking is considered resistance exercise but for today, get a bit more creative. Add lunges during walks for a great modification, or find a set of stairs to intermix with your cardio. Another simple suggestion is to perform calf raises, wall sits, squats, or squat jumps, depending on your level. Mix these into walking or another form of heart- pumping exercise. I recommend seven minutes of cardio, followed by three minutes of resistance based, done a minimum of three times for a total of thirty minutes.

D.I.E.T. #101

Use your body weight to change up your exercise today. Remember, the more weight you have the harder it is, but the more benefit you will get from it.

April 11

Eat more vegetables. You've heard it a thousand times, and you know they are good for you. Now how in the world can you incorporate more? If you aren't a big fan of them, veggies are hard to eat at every meal. So how about a larger serving, each time you eat them?

A normal sized salad has two servings of vegetables because it contains two cups of volume. The recommendation for vegetables is to eat two and a half servings each day. Consider adding more to your salad and you will meet the daily veggie requirement! Choose a greens and veggie based salad for your main course, then add toppings such as grilled meats, nuts, seeds, roasted veggies, and oil based dressing.

D.I.E.T. #102

Eat a salad today. Measure it to include two and a half cups of vegetables, and add protein and healthy fat based toppings to balance out your meal.

April 12

Relaxing is hard to do with so many other priorities. It might seem crazy to prioritize it, but making sure you do it is so important that today is devoted to doing something that physically relaxes the body. When done consistently, lowering stress hormones through relaxation can contribute to weight loss and overall health.

Warmth helps loosen tight muscles and encourages blood flow. Warming up also requires the body to cool down, which is why after a long hot shower you may feel tired. In the morning, I suggest quick showers, but in the evening prior to bed, taking a warm bath can help you relax and sleep better. Soaking in the tub doesn't have to take a long time, if you focus on clearing your mind and spending your time without distraction.

D.I.E.T. #103

Take a bath. If you don't have a bathtub, take a long shower and add a scented body wash or something you don't normally take time for. Do this before bed to help you relax and fall asleep faster.

April 13

Eating the same foods in smaller portions helps people lose weight due to reduction in total calories consumed. Of course it works best with healthy foods, but for today, simply bring awareness to the portion sizes you typically eat.

What is the difference between serving size and portion? A portion is what you consume, while a serving is what is suggested or on the label (if your food has one). Make note of the suggested serving size on any packaged food you eat, compared to the size you typically consume. In general, use the size of your palm for a suggested protein serving, and a small handful for starches like rice and healthy fats like nuts. A fresh fruit serving is the size of a baseball. Remember the suggested serving size for non-starchy vegetables is unlimited!

D.I.E.T. #104

Compare serving sizes to your portion sizes. This exercise brings awareness to whether you may be overeating, and can help in your efforts to feel better and lose weight, if that is your goal.

April 14

The Internet can have a negative impact on people who attempt weight loss. Images, ideas, and fads crowd the online spaces that you are likely looking at. Instead of using social media to see what others are doing and how they are succeeding, search health and wellness professional's web-sites for ideas that will work for you.

In the field of exercise, there are many professionals who give free advice through their websites or on various video-based sites. Search for exercise physiologists, physical therapists, or certified personal trainers who offer workouts to guide you. Depending on your level, choose a workout routine you can follow until it gets easier. This could be stretching, yoga, or interval style. Once you are ready for the next challenge, progress to the next level or the next professional.

D.I.E.T. #105

Use the computer for exercise inspiration today. Search for a professional who offers online or video based coaching.

April 15

In addition to remembering today as "tax day," use today to reflect on the sacrifices and choices you have made for your health. Have they added up and paid you back yet? Having the discipline to make choices that are good for your body and mind is possible, and when you make good choices, your sense of self-control improves.

Recognize that you won't make the right choice every time, but every choice you make pushes you in one direction or the other. Little things add up, and small mistakes won't crumble you! Today, keep accumulating good choices. Notice the refund you get, both immediately, and in the near future.

D.I.E.T. #106

Today, notice the refund you are getting from hard work, and celebrate it by speaking a few positive words to yourself. If you just started, and you aren't seeing a refund yet this year, remember it is coming!

April 16

Eating smaller portions, eating different foods, and eating at different times are all ways to change up your diet. Today's D.I.E.T. involves considering the way you prepare your meal, in addition to planning what foods you will cook.

Fried foods are the obvious answer when someone asks the question "What should I avoid at a restaurant?" This applies to a home cooked meal as well. In addition, using baking and broiling versus pan cooking, boiling, and frying will help reduce fat content, and can help retain more nutrients. Grilling is another way to lower fat content, but make sure you are using low fat skinless cuts, and avoiding heavy gravies, butter, and other toppings.

D.I.E.T. #107

Use the oven or grill instead of another method today. You'll save yourself some calories and unhealthy fat grams. Consider adding veggies to your baking dish or grill for extra roasted flavors.

April 17

Are eggs good, or are they bad? They are good! Yes, the 2015-2020 dietary guidelines suggest limiting saturated fat to 10% of daily calories, but do not specify a limit to cholesterol intake. Eggs are one of those tricky foods that have cholesterol, but not a lot of saturated fat, so they can be eaten along with other sources of protein, as often as on a daily basis.

I won't hold back. Eggs are my favorite breakfast food. If I don't eat them, I am hungry by mid-morning, and I snack in the afternoon. It's a proven personal experiment! Plus, they taste good for breakfast, or any other meal for that matter. My favorite way to cook them is over-medium, and I think the tastiest way to eat them is over a piece of toast smeared with avocado. Yum!

D.I.E.T. #108

Have eggs for breakfast to celebrate my birthday. I'm certainly going to join you!

April 18

Processed foods are foods that have been changed from their naturally occurring state. Oils are not an exception. Sometimes their chemical structure is changed to make them more appealing in the production and stability of packaged foods. Processed "trans" fats are harmful to your heart. Avoiding foods in boxes will help you avoid oils that have been chemically altered to improve their shelf stability.

Another way to avoid these oils is to avoid foods that contain the word "hydrogenated" on their ingredient list. Naturally occurring trans fats are consumed in dairy and animal products, and in small amounts, these are not considered dangerous. However, "hydrogenated" oils have been changed from a liquid to a solid state by altering their chemical structure, and should be avoided.

D.I.E.T. #109

Today, avoid eating foods with hydrogenated oils. In addition, take a pantry inventory and get rid of any packaged foods that have hydrogenated on the ingredient label.

April 19

Getting more nutrients from natural foods is something I'm totally into. However, it has to taste good and be satisfying too. Texture is a big part of it for me. I like crunch, and one way to achieve a big crunch is to add chia seeds to a healthy snack.

Whether you like sweet or salty, chia seeds work. Add them to sweet snacks like flavored Greek yogurt or your favorite protein-containing energy bites. Or, try chia pudding by mixing 2 cups of your favorite milk with 1/2 of a cup of chia seeds and 1½ cups smashed berries. Let it sit in the fridge for at least 4 hours, then eat as is, or choose toppings like shredded coconut, chocolate shavings, or crushed nuts.

D.I.E.T. #110

Make something with chia seeds today. They are full of omega 3 fats, fiber, and crunch to satisfy and provide you with long lasting energy.

April 20

Sometimes being an adult isn't much fun. It's possible to act like a child in some of the things we do, especially when it comes to exercise. As a kid, playing outside and being in gym class was fun, likely because it involved games. It can still be fun to exercise! Whether you do it as an interval-style workout with fun props, or you try some of the following moves, incorporate a game-like attitude about your activity.

Try animal themed exercises. The following activities get your whole body involved and don't require equipment! Bear Crawl involves walking on all fours across the room and back. Frog jumps are repeated big jumps forward. Crab walk is walking backwards on hands and feet, and is great for the arms. Try cat-cow stretching for a cool down core exercise. Try these exercises in the middle of your cardio routine, or on their own.

D.I.E.T. #111

Exercise like an animal today. A few sets and you'll wear yourself out!

April 21

Sitting for long periods of time has been compared to smoking, in terms of its harmfulness to your health. It doesn't surprise me, but it seems like a real downer for people who like to sit on the couch after dinner. We sit enough on the job, driving, at children's activities, and even while doing productive things like sending a friend an email or talking on the phone.

To avoid sitting is not realistic, but to take away a seated activity that is unproductive and unnecessary can certainly help! If you are going to take one thing away, consider television. I'm not saying forever, but for one day. If you focus on meal planning or core exercise and are sitting, that is productive. If you are working, that is necessary. Even though I love to watch my favorite shows, I know it isn't productive OR necessary. Give your body a break today!

D.I.E.T. #112

Avoid watching TV. It's might not be easy, but it's a simple, direct, and helpful D.I.E.T. for today!

April 22

Making your plate colorful doesn't happen without some planning. If you don't think much, a meal can end up very white and tan! It might take some thought, but the vitamins and minerals in bright foods, along with other whole-body healthy compounds make including color well worth it!

Orange is a color that in veggies, generally indicates beta-carotene or Vitamin A, while in fruits, may suggest Vitamin C. In cheese, well, that's another story. Choose a serving of orange colored fruits or vegetables to include in at least one meal today. A whole source is preferred, over juices made of fruits and veggies. The less processing and more natural the food, the better your body can utilize its benefits. Some of my favorite orange foods are salmon, a small sweet potato, baby carrots, cantaloupe, or a clementine. Get creative and colorful today!

D.I.E.T. #113

Eat something orange today. Have at least one serving. And sorry, but macaroni and cheese doesn't count!

April 23

The urge to eat can be brought on by many things other than actual hunger. Sometimes the need to chew something or have fresh breath drives a craving. Instead of giving in right away, turn on your hunger gauge and decide if you are truly hungry. If not, try chewing on something harmless, such as a piece of gum.

Personally, artificial sweeteners in gum irritate my stomach, as do colorings such as red dye. So, I've found that chewing a white piece of gum or a soft mint works well when it's freshness that I'm craving, not food. If you're going to a meeting or to a place where gum is inappropriate, opt for the mint, or even just a few seconds of chewing gum. Just make sure you have a tissue to spit it out, instead of having to swallow it!

D.I.E.T. #114

Use chewing gum to stave off a craving. For the record, it doesn't take seven years to digest if you swallow it, but try to find a place to spit it out if you are headed into a place where chewing might be inappropriate.

April 24

A strategy many people use for weight loss is to buy clothing that they want to fit into, or to pull out an old pair of jeans that have become too small. While this is a great way to motivate some, it can also be helpful to go ahead and *wear* something a bit tight.

It is not torture that I am suggesting, but giving yourself a gentle reminder throughout the day to eat smaller portions of foods that make you feel good. These reminders will keep your pants or top from pulling across the midsection, and will keep you feeling confident and strong in your willpower.

D.I.E.T. #115

Wear something you feel slightly uncomfortable in. Not only does it probably look better than you think, but wearing something a bit snug will give you posture reminders and remind you to eat better throughout the day. This will help keep your mind and body strong!

April 25

There are many ways to slow down, and while it may seem silly to count, remember that counting is one way to delay a reaction. As a child, you likely heard, "I'm going to count to three...." This is an example of someone delaying a reaction by giving a warning for unruly behavior. Similarly, counting to three before you eat, or better yet to ten, can give you a moment to remember that eating is not a race.

Taking a ten second pause prior to beginning a meal or snack can be a silent or out-loud strategy. Adding this behavior before every eating event will very likely improve your feelings about food, at least for today. It will help you relax, and can be very effective when trying to separate eating from emotion.

D.I.E.T. #116

Count to ten before you begin eating. Say it in your head, or say it out loud, but purposefully counting at least a few numbers prior to eating is a great experiment for today.

April 26

Quality sleep can make or break you. Most people need seven to nine hours of sleep, but it isn't all about the hours if you aren't getting quality time. Resetting and recovering is what sleep is all about, and it is a critical part of our health.

Relaxing before bed can help get you off to dreamland faster, and will help you stay asleep longer. Besides turning off the television sooner, try having something to drink before bed. Give yourself twenty minutes prior to bedtime to sip something warm. Then, you can use the bathroom and empty your bladder before falling asleep. If you tolerate milk, it can help melatonin levels, but if you don't, try herbal tea or warm water with a squeeze of lemon. The warmth can calm and soothe, and can also help your bowels in the morning.

D.I.E.T. #117

Have a warm drink before bed. It is typically the soothing warmth versus magic ingredients that calm a person to sleep.

April 27

It is hard enough to get motivated for today, so when I suggest doing something for tomorrow, many people don't welcome the request for extra effort! However, if I could give a suggestion that is no more work for today and would benefit you tomorrow, would you accept the challenge?

Whether you are whipping up a casserole for dinner, have meat ready for the grill, or are making soup in the slow cooker, it's simple enough to make extra. Double the recipe and when it is done, cover in a separate container, chop into usable leftover portions, or divide into lunch size containers. There's the extra work, but it is minimal and will save you tomorrow, and possibly in the days to come.

D.I.E.T. #118

Make a meal for tomorrow, today! It could also be for next week, or for a friend. Depending on your needs, make a meal for a time that would otherwise be stressful or become takeout.

April 28

Weaving exercise into your day might sound complicated and sweaty, but it doesn't have to be. For example, if I told you to stand up right now and do 10 jumping jacks, you could do some form of this without a problem, and without breaking a sweat. Getting up from a seated position and moving is an overwhelmingly popular suggestion, for good reason!

No matter what you are doing during the day, interrupting it with a burst of exercise when your body doesn't expect it can create some appealing effects. Effects such as increased breathing, enhanced focus, improved mood, and a boost in energy.

D.I.E.T. #119

This one might sound awful, but it is really simple. Do jumping jacks. A few times today. They can be any type, even the kind where your feet don't leave the floor. Just wave your arms overhead and step out and in. Do it at least ten times, and repeat at least three times today.

April 29

When we speak positively, our lives follow. A genuinely loving attitude changes everything. Sometimes it isn't easy to force yourself into positivity, so for today, try the following strategy: speak the words you want to believe over and over again. Maybe you don't believe it at all yet, maybe you know that person is deep within, or maybe you do believe it. It doesn't matter. Today is about positivity.

Speak about strength, self-control, kindness, and happiness. Decide who it is you are (or want to become) and say it out loud. Don't limit this to just one time today. Say it over and over, and act upon it whenever you see an opportunity today.

D.I.E.T. #120

Say you are who you want to be. I am strong. I am in control. I am likeable. Building your own self-esteem is not easy, and it takes lots of practice, but it is critical to your success.

April 30

One thing that helps me in multiple aspects of my health is stretching. Some people don't believe in the value of stretching, possibly because they don't do it enough. They say, "it doesn't help," or "it hurts too much." These reasons are precisely why you should do it more!

The most helpful time to stretch, in my experience, is before bed. It is the most efficient too, because it not only helps flexibility and joint pain, but it can aid in relaxation and a better night of sleep. Do two to three simple stretches, one at a time, holding each for twenty or more seconds and then repeating the stretch.

D.I.E.T. #121

Stretch before bed. I suggest a toe-touch stretch and a chest opening stretch such as lying back with arms overhead or out to the sides. A gentle twist, knees to one side and then the other is helpful too, to ease lower back pain.

May 1

Today marks one third of the way through the year, so let's talk about dividing up calories. Calories come from carbohydrate, protein, and fat. Often times it isn't the amount of food eaten, but the kinds that keep us from achieving better health. So today, aim to eat one third of your calories from protein, one third from carbohydrate, and one third from fat.

Use a tracking tool to make it easier. There are many apps that are easy to use. If you're not a techy person, here's how to do the math. Take your total number of calories and divide by 3. For a carb and protein grams goal, divide again by 4 (since there are 4 calories per gram of each). For your fat goal, divide by 9 (there are 9 calories per gram of fat). Then, enter your food intake and aim to achieve those numbers.

D.I.E.T. #122

Focus on thirds. This activity helps you think of food more scientifically. It might be more time consuming than other strategies, but you will learn a lot, and you might decide to do it more often!

May 2

For the 123rd day of the year, remember that practicing something hard eventually makes it as easy as 1, 2, 3. It makes sense to practice things that are challenging, yet achievable, as these things will get easier with time. The easier they get, the more motivated you will be to press on toward more difficult goals. It is important to be patient and consistent, practicing things that take time to improve, then moving on.

I'll use the example goal of walking around the block. For some, this may take working on walking to the mailbox everyday, and progressing toward walking down the street before getting the mail. Eventually that will be easy, and walking around the block will be the goal. For others, a marathon may be the long- term vision, and today is the 5K jog. Keep your eyes set on the 1, 2, 3 goal for today, but remember your future goal too.

D.I.E.T. #123

Practice something you think is challenging today, and watch it become easy as 1,2,3.

May 3

If it doesn't feel like spring yet, get out the grill. Making something fresh on the grill can set you up for a healthy day. In the morning, get your fish, meat, or chicken defrosting, and take the grill cover off, so you are sure to come home and use it! If you want to go meatless, prepare some quick black bean burgers or plan to pick up some Portobello mushrooms or fresh veggies to roast.

To make black bean burgers, mash a regular sized can of drained beans with one egg, a teaspoon each of cumin, garlic powder, and chili powder. Add breadcrumbs until patties can be formed. This is a quick and easy grill item, but make sure you oil the grill or use cooking spray to coat your patties and avoid a sticky mess.

D.I.E.T. #124

Use the grill. If you haven't already, it's time to start barbecuing! It doesn't have to be difficult, and keeping your ingredients simple will encourage you to repeat this healthy cooking method again, very soon.

May 4

Avoiding all screens is almost impossible, especially if you work. Still, limiting less useful screen time is great for mental health and energy levels. What is less useful? That depends on you, but it does take a bit of honesty and attention to how much you are looking at your phone, computer, television, and other devices. Chances are, it is more than you think.

There are many people who conduct their business using devices with screens. However, there is likely a lot of time spent on these devices, in addition to what is required for a job. For today, take out non-essential social media and emails. Avoid movies and television. It can wait!

D.I.E.T. #125

Limit all unnecessary screen time. This takes honesty and thoughtfulness. Consider it a mental health day, since it will offer added relaxation time and potentially less screen related "brain fog."

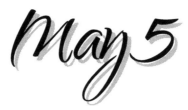

May 5

Simple swapping is a great way to change habits. Eat this, not that was a strategy that became popular because of achievability. One of the simplest swaps that can make a major impact on your health is changing out refined, or white grains for whole varieties.

Eating more whole grains doesn't have to mean whole wheat everything. A great whole grain to include is quinoa. Try making this swap today, changing out rice, pasta, or potato choices for a simple side dish. Quinoa is it's own grain and is easy to make. Cook it like you would rice on the stovetop, with double the liquid to quinoa ratio. Use stock or broth, or add citrus juice after it's finished. Quinoa will take the flavor of the cooking liquid, or whatever is added.

D.I.E.T. #126

Have a half-cup serving of quinoa today. Cook it ahead of time in a double batch if you prefer. Keep it in the fridge for up to a week to eat as a quick side dish. There are many varieties of quinoa, and endless ways to prepare it if you decide to get creative!

May 6

Most homes have some kind of pantry whether it is a cupboard system, one you designate for snacks, or an entire room. Today is a great day to be a bit critical of your pantry. It's time for a spring cleanup!

Food that is kept in the cupboard almost always has a label. That doesn't always mean it is unhealthy, but it probably means it is easy to snack on. Set aside ten to twenty minutes today to purge some of the less healthy items. First, toss anything that has hydrogenated on the ingredient label. Next, look for sugars in the double digits. Last but not least, be honest with foods you eat when emotional, foods that cause you to overeat, or foods that you consider triggers. Toss them! Replace with items like nuts, single serve or portioned snacks, rice cakes, popcorn, and whole grains that can be cooked quickly.

D.I.E.T. #127

Clean out your pantry! If you have a large space full of snacks, you may have to spend more time, but it will be worth it.

May 7

Should you eat three square meals, or four to six small meals and snacks? It's a long debated question. The answer is, it probably doesn't matter that much. What does matter is finding a pattern you can stick to, and eating at purposeful times. Otherwise it becomes "grazing," which I define as snacking all day without clear start and end times.

Commit to eating just three times today. Determine what you will eat at each meal that contains protein, whole grain carbs, and a fruit or vegetable. Have a plan for what you need to accomplish after you finish, so you can avoid grazing. When you are finished, wait at least three hours until you eat again. If you want to space meals evenly, you would eat them approximately 5 hours apart (assuming eight hours of rest).

D.I.E.T. #128

Skip snacks today. Limit yourself to three balanced and evenly spaced meals. Finish dinner at least three hours before bedtime.

May 8

I love the idea that life is a sum of all of your choices. I often suggest visualizing a spectrum of success, with one end signifying total failure and the other end accomplishing a long-term goal. The next part takes believing that every choice moves you only one step. Remember that your lifetime is full of millions of choices, and every day is full of hundreds of healthy or unhealthy moves.

Forward or backward, you are moving one spot with each choice. Doughnut for breakfast-- one move back. Healthy salad with lunch-- one move forward. Skipping the office snacks-- one move forward. Remember that your day's choices will accumulate, and the goal is to end up in a positive direction.

D.I.E.T. #129

Set a ruler on your kitchen counter, to remember the spectrum of success. Remind yourself that every choice matters. Make more healthy choices and you will move more quickly toward your goal.
In addition, you will realize you can overcome a mistake, or poor choice.

May 9

Getting the body moving is important for metabolism, but becoming less sedentary is step one. You don't have to perform exhausting workouts every day. Physical activity means anything beyond resting, which means cleaning, walking around the house, getting the mail or shopping all fit! If you don't have the stamina for cleaning and shopping, there are other ways to add to your day.

All of these things qualify as Non-exercise Activity Thermogenesis. "N.E.A.T." are calories burned by physical activity that isn't structured exercise. It even includes doing simple things like standing while talking on the phone, or tapping your fingers and toes while sitting. The more an activity makes you work, the more benefit you will get from it. Thinking of it this way, N.E.A.T. is a friendly addition to your activity level.

D.I.E.T. #130

Use N.E.A.T. for added activity today. Take a pet for a walk or pick a parking spot farther away. It doesn't have to be complicated!

May 10

It's hard to deny that music makes everyone feel good, and when moving about, music can naturally increase the tempo of your steps. Jogging to a specific beat, or singing along to your favorite tunes makes the time go by faster, may keep you from thinking about the exertion, and can encourage a higher intensity of exercise.

Listening to the radio is one way to do it, but listening to a list of your favorite tunes can be exhilarating and fun. Commercials and commentary can be aggravating when listening to the radio so I suggest regularly reorganizing a playlist. Include a mixture of old and new upbeat music. Consider a fresh song purchase for your playlist as a reward for reaching a certain milestone during the week.

D.I.E.T. #131

Organize or create a playlist for exercise. If you owe yourself a reward, add a new song. You'll be surprised how refreshing it can be to your workout routine.

May 11

By now, spring has likely produced some color outside. If you are fortunate enough to have plants and flowers in your yard, they are a wonderful way to spruce up your eating environment. As you have probably noticed, a lightened mood can translate into healthier eating, so create a space that is cheerful using home grown color.

Take advantage of your flowerbeds or pots, or make a quick stop at the store for some fresh cut flowers. If you have allergies, daffodils, geranium, and crocus are some of the best, as are roses and tulips. Find a simple vase or jar and place them on your table. Enjoy them while you are eating, and thank yourself for bringing the colors of spring inside!

D.I.E.T. #132

Put flowers on your table. Creating a positive environment is important in relaxing, appreciating, and enjoying mealtime. It can also help you slow down your eating, to "enjoy the roses," of course!

May 12

Learning to appreciate and respect food for what it provides to your body is important. Living with gratitude can affect the food choices you make, the activities you commit to, the relationships you are involved in, and the way you choose to spend your time.

Being grateful for food should include being genuinely thankful for the nourishment and enjoyment it provides. This gratitude makes eating more purposeful, and can prevent the use of food as a coping mechanism. In addition, being thankful in general can remind us where true happiness is found. Being grateful for a body that functions well can bring us to exercise more often, and being thankful for family may encourage us to prioritize a home cooked meal to share together.

D.I.E.T. #133

Write down five things you are grateful for. This exercise will encourage you to stay positive and to share this contagious joy with others.

May 13

I once had a client with an addiction to crust-less sandwiches. If she's reading this, she knows. All foods can fit into a healthy diet, but certain feelings around the food can make it unhealthy. An addiction or out of control feeling around any food suggests it may be helpful to dig deeper into your connection with this food.

How do you know if you have an addiction or strange behavior related to a specific food? It is likely easy to know, but often it's hard to admit. If you can't avoid buying a certain food, consistently eat more than one serving, crave it often, or see it as "bad," it is likely a trigger food, eaten when feeling certain emotions.

D.I.E.T. #134

Admit a strange feeling or secret addiction. Tell someone, and then take action to avoid connecting emotion with this food. You may have to remove it from your house temporarily, or have someone else do it.

May 14

Most of us expect rewards from hard work. Do a good job at work, get a raise; exercise more, lose weight. When trying to lose weight or be healthier, the end goal isn't typically on the timeline we want it to be. So plug in your choice of rewards along the way, rewards that you will really enjoy. In addition to choosing the prizes, you also get to pick the timeline that will best motivate you.

I like to suggest mini rewards on a weekly or every other week basis. My personal favorite is new music for my playlist, but I also love a new pair of running socks or an iced coffee from my favorite shop. For reaching a longer-term goal, a new apparel item or piece of jewelry is a good motivator. A manicure or something else I don't normally make time for also qualifies as a non-food reward.

D.I.E.T. #135

Think about a reward for a long-term goal you are working toward. Choose a mini goal to help you reach the long-term goal, and determine when and what you will do to reward yourself.

May 15

A scale is not discussed much in D.I.E.T.S. 365, because healthy goals are better measured with something other than weight. Weight loss may be the end result of changed habits, but try focusing on results other than weight, such as body shape.

Waist circumference is directly related to disease risk, so from an overall health standpoint it is the most important place to lose fat from. I suggest using a belt to measure your success. A tape measure can also do the trick, but if you want to gauge success without using numbers, try a belt instead. Measure what hole you are using now, and choose a hole you would realistically like to achieve. Then, make mini goals toward it. Make sure you are taking your belt loop assessment consistently in the morning, when bloating is at a minimum, and don't expect results day to day. Try measuring every two to four weeks.

D.I.E.T. #136

Cinch up a belt buckle. To reach a smaller waist circumference, it will take consistent steps forward with your diet and exercise. So keep reading and making daily changes!

May 16

Once you start something, it is typically easier to keep going. The law of inertia says an object in motion continues in motion with the same speed and in the same direction unless acted upon. This is the same as with exercise. Get the momentum to start and inertia will take over. Then you can add five minutes instead of struggle with getting started.

Try this. Go into your exercise with a specific duration in mind. It doesn't matter if it's thirty minutes of walking or five minutes of abdominal exercises, but get started. When you reach the end of your workout, tell yourself to continue for five more minutes. Your next commitment can wait for five more minutes, especially when you are feeling good.

D.I.E.T. #137

Add five more minutes. It can be additional minutes of the same activity, or you could choose something such as stretching or cooling down. Once you try this, you'll see how easy it is to workout for just a bit longer!

May 17

If you are exhausted by the time you get to bed, you might have a big pile of nightstand books waiting to be finished. However, a book that is short, or devotional style can provide a lot of bang per word. A paragraph can do a lot of good when read before heading off to sleep.

Sometimes devotionals are seen as morning routines, but there is equal use for them at night. Getting relaxed and reading something calming is helpful, or pick something motivational to end your day on a positive note. Don't just read your favorite romance novel, though that could also distract your mind from stress! Read something that will stick with you through the night and help you wake up refreshed. The mind does creative things during sleep, so relaxing prior to bed can help you wake up refreshed and ready for a productive day.

D.I.E.T. #138

Read something helpful before bed tonight. It doesn't have to be D.I.E.T.S. 365, but it could be!

May 18

Athletes typically stick to a routine and eat healthy foods because they know it makes a difference. If an athlete is a professional or has a scholarship, it is a priority to win, which requires peak performance. Everything must be done to guarantee top results. This includes regularly spaced meals, fueling for workouts and careful attention to hydration.

Fueling your body can be more easily prioritized when you are active, but even if you can't exercise you can understand how healthy eating is necessary for feeling your best. Start by eating fresh foods and avoiding extra sugar. Treat yourself to regularly spaced meals of high quality foods for ideal energy production. Hydrate with water for better focus.

D.I.E.T. #139

Think about eating like an athlete would. Pretend to be an athlete if you have to, and believe that you are fueling your body for today's performance! It will remind you to stay on track.

May 19

We are more likely to eat new or healthier foods when they are flavored with familiar, or exciting ingredients. If you serve plain cooked green beans, it won't be as enjoyable as if you top them with lemon pepper and almond slices.

Flavoring fresh vegetables and proteins with herbs is a way to bring more satisfaction to your meals. Take it a step further and buy the herbs from a farmer's market, or pot your own to use over and over. Examples of easy to grow herbs include basil, dill, and mint. Try a new spin on basil by using Thai or purple varieties, and if you are able to find fresh cilantro or oregano, try those instead of dried varieties.

D.I.E.T. #140

Use a new spice or herb. If you only have dried herbs on hand, it's ok, but make sure they are not expired! Try sage on poultry or on butternut squash, turmeric in rice dishes, or rosemary on roasted vegetables.

May 20

Feeling good makes a person look good, and looking good makes a person feel good. It's true that the two go hand in hand. So which comes first? Start by trying something that helps you look good, such as dressing up a bit more today. Depending on what is on the calendar, this could mean fixing your hair instead of wearing a hat, or it might be high heels instead of flats.

Now that you are looking good, pay attention to how you feel! Notice if you make better choices overall when you take pride in your appearance. Don't worry if you get compliments or not, and avoid people who might ask, "Why are you all dressed up today?" You don't owe anyone an explanation, unless you *want* to share.

D.I.E.T. #141

Get dressed up today. Be proud of yourself, and let your pride carry you through a strong and healthy day!

May 21

Variety is important in your diet, and mixing up your exercise routine is helpful as well. Not only can it trick your body into burning more calories and losing weight, it can also trick your mind! The mind is likely the only thing stopping you from accomplishing what you want to get done today.

There is a certain route I like to take when running, and when I'm not feeling motivated, I reverse the route. Somehow, it changes things up enough to get me through it. Maybe it is that I don't know the mile markers, or maybe it's the angle of the sun, but it certainly makes me feel better. Is there a park nearby that you could walk through? Or if it's raining, is there an indoor mall you could stroll around to fight off boredom and procrastination of exercise?

D.I.E.T. #142

Take a walk or go jogging somewhere new, or pick a new direction. Doing something different will refresh you and keep you motivated to continue a daily exercise pattern.

May 22

The definition of a super food is one that is rich in nutrients and considered beneficial for health. "Super foods" play a variety of roles in a person's well being. One such food is the delicious avocado!

A ripe avocado is dark purple and gives just a bit to slight pressure. If you purchase them green or unripe, just set them on the counter for a few days. Avocados are full of heart healthy monounsaturated fats, fiber, potassium, and B vitamins. They are a great substitute for butter spread on toast or sandwiches, and are awesome topped with cottage cheese or an over-easy egg.

D.I.E.T. #143

Eat an avocado today. Try this amazing lightened guacamole dip: Place equal portions of pitted peeled avocado and cottage cheese in a good blender. Add a few tablespoons of green salsa and a squeeze of lime. If you like cilantro or parsley, add that too. Blend well, dip with raw veggies, or use on tacos or toast!

May 23

There are so many ways to switch up your eating environment. When you need a night free of dishes, or need to get away from work over lunch, consider packing a disposable picnic. This offers a change to your scenery and can offer a temporary distraction from the usual routine.

Pack a lunch bag with a simple wrap or salad, a whole piece of fruit, nuts or seeds, and an extra protein such as string cheese or a hard cooked egg. If there isn't a table to eat at, bring a towel or blanket to sit on, and take your meal outside. If it's raining, consider heading to a coffee shop and purchase a drink to enjoy with your meal. Be sure to sit by a window!

D.I.E.T. #144

Pack a picnic lunch or dinner. You don't have to eat outdoors, but the idea of a picnic, packed in a different container, can allow you to eat more mindfully. If you choose to enjoy your evening meal this way, avoid dishes by using recyclable paper products.

May 24

Physical and mental balance can be trained together, and improving them simultaneously is a great benefit of exercise. To get the results, you must put in the proper work, so consider adding a balance exercise to your routine today.

A stability ball is a large inflatable ball that supports your body weight. Simply sitting on it can be a challenge, but using it to perform a plank, or holding it up in the air and tilting side to side are also great challenges. You could also choose to stand on one foot while holding the ball between your hands, arms extended straight in front of you. Press into the ball while balancing for as long as you can, and then switch legs.

D.I.E.T. #145

Use a stability ball or practice balancing exercises today. You could do the above activities without a ball, or look up a series of yoga balancing poses. To balance your mind at the same time, notice your breathing while completing the exercise. Try to slow your thoughts as much as possible.

May 25

Breakfast is always easier than dinner, isn't it? I often forget that when there isn't a dinner plan, making breakfast foods is a simple quick option. Sometimes protein is challenging, but here are some ideas to get you considering morning foods again at night!

Choose from one or more of my favorite breakfast proteins: eggs, turkey sausage, ham, bacon (choose a no nitrates variety), tofu scramble, Greek yogurts, milk, cheese, protein pancakes or other items made with protein powders. Decide on an entree such as baked eggs (add fresh spinach) or avocado on toast with an egg, and add sides such as fruit and nuts over Greek yogurt. Or, try oats cooked on the stovetop with protein powder mixed in after cooking.

D.I.E.T. #146

Make breakfast for dinner. Kids typically love having breakfast twice, so I'm not sure why I don't do it more often! Even without kids, it is an easy quick solution to the problem "what's for dinner?"

May 26

The way food looks is a big part of the experience of eating. The sense of sight is utilized before the sense of taste, so give yourself a better chance at enjoyment by adding a little something to your plate. Even if it's a simple meal you are eating alone, adding a garnish is easy and can add to your satisfaction.

My favorite easy garnish is a green sprinkle of something, such as parsley or cilantro. A lemon wedge or other type of fruit also works well to brighten the dish and sweeten the flavor, depending on what you are eating. Mint, edible flowers, or cucumbers are pretty and add color to your dish or to your ice water.

D.I.E.T. #147

Use garnish. If you don't have one, I suggest purchasing a shaker container such as a small glass jar with shaker lid. You can buy fresh garnish to use, and keep the rest to dry. Then add to your container. It takes an extra step up front, but can make a big difference. Dried herbs last a long time, so use them over and over!

May 27

It is widely known that people with high blood pressure should limit their sodium intake, but it is also wise for those with normal blood pressure to avoid excessive salt intake. Salt, the main dietary source of sodium, causes increased stress on the blood vessels, which over the long term can lead to heart disease.

A diet high in sodium also causes water retention and bloating, and can prevent accurate results on a scale. The first step in reducing your salt intake is to stop using table salt in cooking, and over foods. There are many other ways to reduce sodium in the diet such as choosing fresh over canned foods and limiting high sodium dairy, but depending on how much you currently use a salt shaker, eliminating it can make a huge impact.

D.I.E.T. #148

Hide the salt shaker. Whether for blood pressure, weight control, or overall health reasons, reducing sodium in the diet starts with avoiding the addition of salt to your food.

May 28

It is said that "Buddha," who founded Buddhism, was an enlightened soul who had found complete happiness. His tummy was round, likely as he was full and satisfied! It's why I love the name "Buddha Bowl" to describe a layered meal in a bowl.

If you have a few items, a Buddha Bowl is so simple and quick to put together. Start with a whole grain on the bottom. My favorites are brown rice or quinoa, but you can use whole grain pasta, farro, barley, or whatever you have! Veggies are the next layer, so try broccoli, spinach, cauliflower, carrots, or a mix of your favorites. Then add a protein such as grilled chicken, shrimp, beef, tofu, tempeh, or edamame. Top with a sauce. Salsas or hot sauces work well, as do teriyakis, guacamole, oil based dressings, or peanut butter based sauces.

D.I.E.T. #149

Create a Buddha bowl today. Write down exchanges you might make to vary your recipe, and plan to make another version again soon!

May 29

I'm not a huge fan of skipping meals, but sometimes it is an interesting experiment to see if you can go without eating for a few hours. It can also be helpful if you know in advance that you are going to be eating a large meal later in the day.

It is not, however, a good idea to think of it as saving calories in order to binge later. If thought of as restriction in order to "cheat" later, it can turn into an unhealthy cycle. Instead, think about being in better control of your choices throughout the day as to make room for some potential "errors" later! This still takes willpower, and the realization that you can do it is pretty empowering.

D.I.E.T. #150

Save room for dinner. Don't starve yourself, but eat smaller meals and avoid snacking. Plan ahead for a bigger dinner tonight, or save this entry for a day when you have big plans and can put this strategy to good use.

May 30

I like to get ahead of my game, mostly because I don't like to stress out at the last minute. Sometimes getting ahead can seem like a lot of effort, but think of it as over-preparing. You'll be able to get in front of your game, which means you won't have to race at the end.

This concept is helpful to think about when trying to improve your hydration. There are many ways to stay hydrated throughout the day, but if you get off to a slow start, it is much harder to catch up. So, take my "get ahead" mentality and apply it to hydration. Drink water when you first wake up. It might feel like torture trying to drink sixteen ounces before anything else, but trust the process! It can change your day by increasing your focus and energy, helping you to avoid cravings, and keeping you satisfied.

D.I.E.T. #151

Drink sixteen ounces of water when you first wake up, or plan to do it tomorrow morning. When you feel the effects of this, you'll want to do it again and again.

May 31

One year, a friend gave me three of her extra kale plants. After easily potting them, I had leafy greens all summer long. Many people think of salad or steamed kale, but there are lots of uses for this powerhouse vegetable!

Kale chips sound intimidating, but they are a healthy snack that I encourage everyone to try making, because they are simple and provide so much nutritional value for your effort! Here's how:

> Heat your oven to 300. Wash and dry kale, and slice into pieces, avoiding the large vein in the center (if there is one in your variety). Toss kale in a drizzle of olive oil. Lay pieces in one layer on a baking sheet coated with cooking spray. Bake for 20-25 minutes, turning over carefully in the middle of baking. Remove from oven, add seasoning if you like, and enjoy!

D.I.E.T. #152

Bake homemade kale chips. Spritz with vinegar, or add non-salt spices after baking to make them irresistible!

June 1

Grilling is a healthy way to prepare meats and veggies, especially if you take care to avoid excess smoke and charring. HCA and PAH, the compounds that form when cooking meat at high temperatures have been shown to cause cancer. Avoiding excessive production of these compounds takes a bit of care and preparation.

Marinating meat gives it a barrier, prevents smoke from permeating the surface, and helps meat retains its moisture. Using a leaner cut of meat will also keep drips of fat from creating PAH filled smoke. To avoid excessive HCA, turn your meat often, and stop grilling before it is well done. This limits time and heat, which are both necessary for HCA to form.

D.I.E.T. #153

Use lean cuts of meat on the grill today, and practice healthier grilling by marinating, flipping regularly, and skewering, to require less time on the grill.

June 2

Looking forward to something can keep attitudes positive and moods happy. Recently I saw a license plate that read "LIV4VACA" and while I'm not sure I *live* for vacation, I certainly live *better* when I have vacation on my mind. Today, focus on the steps you can take to meet your goals by vacation time.

Being more goal-oriented is definitely easier when there is a reward in sight. If you don't have one booked already, plan a vacation. It could be a short getaway or a weekend with friends. If you can't get out of town, make arrangements for someone to come visit *you*, and then decide on a few special outings. Put the dates on your calendar and plan your long-term goal around this vacation.

D.I.E.T. #154

Focus your efforts around your planned "getaway." Decide what you will accomplish by this date, then keep your eye on the reward of some time away from the normal routine.

June 3

Most people would agree that it is fun to eat. However, if you are finding that food has become a favorite pastime, it might be time to focus on a different hobby. Return to a mindset that reminds you, food is for function! Take up a new activity, or renew your passion for something you had put away.

Doing something distracting when you are feeling hungry is a great idea. Make sure you choose an action that is enjoyable or productive. I often suggest things like starting a load of laundry to put off eating, which isn't necessarily enjoyable, but is certainly productive! Today, try distracting yourself with something actionable, and remember that food isn't the only thing you can get happiness from.

D.I.E.T. #155

Do something you enjoy today. Get outdoors, pick up a good book, or play a game with family. Remember, food doesn't give love, but you can learn to love food in a new way if you adopt the idea that food is purposeful.

June 4

I almost chose this **D.I.E.T.** for my birthday, because it is something I do very regularly. I eat a lot of vegetables, and having something to dress a salad with was is the most important step I took to succeed at the challenge of eating more greens.

Eating a salad on most days of the week will provide the fiber, vitamins, and minerals needed to stay active and energetic, and to maintain a healthy weight. Using homemade salad dressing can provide lots of flavor without all the additives found in premade varieties! Homemade dressing is easy. Make simple vinaigrettes with equal parts olive oil and vinegar, plus a small dollop of Dijon mustard, and herbs of your choice. I choose basil and oregano, then sweeten it with a tiny drizzle of honey.

D.I.E.T. #156

Make homemade salad dressing. Oil based dressings can harden in the refrigerator, so if you make it ahead, take it out a few minutes before serving. Shake it up, top your salad, and enjoy.

June 5

Soup is often thought of as a wintertime staple, but there are soups that are fantastic in the heat of the summer. Refreshing and full of nutrients, soup can be ready in an instant, and will satisfy you without all the bloat of carbohydrate heavy meals.

Try a cold soup during the hot weather, and choose a variety with lots of vegetables. Traditionally, soup served cold is fruit or vegetable based, and cold tomato based varieties are often called gazpacho. To make a fruity option, choose two fruits (the fewer the seeds, the better). Blend two cups of fruit with one cup of vanilla Greek yogurt and one cup of your favorite milk. If you like your soup colder and thicker, freeze the fruit first.

D.I.E.T. #157

Make a cold soup. There are thousands of varieties of gazpacho, and with endless combinations of fruits and veggies, there are thousands of other possibilities too. Make sure your blender is ready for some action!

June 6

Fresh air is invigorating, can change your attitude, and liven up your senses. If you feel the drag of the morning or experience afternoon fogginess, taking a step outside could fix things. A brief breath of air, even if it's hot, can help clear your mind and reset your day.

Try this experiment today. After every time of eating, take a step outside, or open the window if you aren't able to go out. You don't have to stay out longer than it takes to get one or two deep breaths. This actionable step can put you back in control and help you feel a bit more energy than if you were to simply go back to your desk or meeting.

D.I.E.T. #158

Go outside after each meal or snack. For both physiological and mental reasons, breaking up sedentary behaviors will offer you a burst of energy you didn't have before.

June 7

Relaxing isn't something that comes naturally, especially if you are an anxious type of person. Most people realize that relaxation is beneficial, but in a stressful moment, it isn't easy. Learning a specific movement to practice, or position to hold can be a lifesaver through troublesome times.

Even if you know nothing about yoga, you can learn a simple practice to use for relaxing. Child's pose is a commonly used for relaxation, but there are others that can be taken anywhere and can even be done with others around. Consider a seated stretch with arms overhead, or a seated twist. Even if you are sitting in a meeting or around others, you can take a few breaths while focusing on your body. Unless you are doing the talking, it will likely go unnoticed.

D.I.E.T. #159

Learn a yoga pose or simple stretch to practice. Taking your mind off of a stressful moment by focusing on your breath and repositioning your body will help reduce aches, pains, and stress.

June 8

Homemade versions of packaged snacks often taste better than premade varieties. While it takes a bit more time, there are serious benefits to decreasing the quantity of packaged foods you eat. Compare basic tortilla chips to the homemade version, and you will see a decrease in fat of over six grams per serving. Calories are a bit lower in the homemade version, as is sodium.

This recipe is so simple, and the chips end up super crunchy and flavorful! Here's how: Heat your oven to 350 degrees. Stack three thin corn tortillas and use a pizza cutter or sharp knife to cut into four to six triangles, so you end up with twelve to eighteen chips. Spray a baking sheet with cooking spray and lay chips in a single layer. Spray the tops and sprinkle with sea salt or another seasoning such as chili powder or nutritional yeast. Bake four to five minutes, then flip and bake until crispy and golden.

D.I.E.T. #160

Make homemade tortilla chips today. Let them cool a bit, and enjoy with a simple salsa!

June 9

It's especially important to drink extra water in the summer months. It seems to be easier when it's hot to drink fluids, but sometimes water gets boring! If you are someone who gets tired of plain water, make it more interesting by adding some natural flavors.

Consider fruits and vegetables soaked in your water. My favorites are strawberries, citrus fruits, and cucumbers, but you can use whatever you have on hand. Make sure it is organic, and thoroughly washed. A thinly sliced cucumber makes water taste more crisp and refreshing. Floating slices of fruit or berries are other options, and using an infuser style pitcher allows you to have flavors without the chunks! If you cut your berries up a bit, flavors will be disbursed more evenly.

D.I.E.T. #161

Make infused water. A simple floating fruit or veggie works well. Be sure to eat your leftovers when the water is gone!

June 10

Overeating in the afternoon and evening hours can be a difficult habit to overcome. It almost always happens when a person is over-hungry, or is eating for reasons other than hunger. If you are eating as a release from the day, or because you didn't eat enough early on, the approach is the same. To fight the afternoon urges, have a controlled snack before you get home.

A pre-portioned item is best, and it is appropriate to have this snack an hour or so before you get home from your day, or whenever that craving typically comes along. The snack should have protein or healthy fats, and could contain whole grains as well. Protein and fats will help stabilize your blood sugar, which can fall in the late afternoon hours, causing cravings.

D.I.E.T. #162

Have a controlled snack before you get home, mid to late afternoon. Examples include a serving of nuts, an ounce of cheese, a protein based shake, or piece of fruit with nut butter.

June 11

Changing up your routine can help you with motivation and energy. When it comes to breakfast, it is typically recommended as the most important meal of the day. Newer research shows that fasting a bit longer into the morning hours can help blood sugars and energy levels later in the day.

If you have a habit of eating breakfast, it isn't a bad thing! However, skip it today and see how you feel later in the day. Begin eating four to five hours after waking instead of the typical 1-2 hours. It is important to eat the right things when you decide to eat your first meal of the day later. Selecting a whole grain carbohydrate with protein and a bit of healthy fat is critical to helping your body utilize the right fuel for energy.

D.I.E.T. #163

Skip breakfast. If you already do this, eat breakfast instead! The point is to change up your morning routine and see how it affects you. A great "first meal" example is a cooked egg served on a corn tortilla spread with avocado, and topped with salsa.

June 12

When it's hot, outdoor exercise is the last thing you want to do. Change your thought about exercising outdoors in the summer by hopping in the pool! You could do it inside too, if you belong to an area rec center or gym that doesn't have one outdoors.

If you aren't a great swimmer, walking in the pool is amazing body weight exercise, and you'll work up a sweat without feeling sweaty! Aqua jogging is another option, and swimming laps is a great calorie burner. If you have kids, playing can disguise the exercise involved. Tossing kids in the water, pulling them on rafts and throwing balls while you jump up and down in the water are all ways to turn up the heat without feeling it!

D.I.E.T. #164

Get in the water! Find a public pool to head to when the heat is on. It's easier to relax when you're cool from the water, so splash around as long as possible.

June 13

Recycling and reusing is a fantastic daily habit. Today, however, I'm giving you the green light to use disposable dishes. It is an effort to make eating at home easier, and to allow a more casual take on cooking.

Sometimes the best reason for eating out is to avoid the cleanup, so using disposables will help if you are stressed out or tired from a long day. Use one paper plate and only the plastic silverware you need, to avoid excess waste. Bake a casserole in a foil pan, or steam veggies in a disposable steam bag. You can even use steam bags for proteins such as chicken. To avoid serving bowls, dish your meals right on the plate.

D.I.E.T. #165

Skip the dishes today and use disposable and recyclable products instead. Prepare others in the household by telling them you won't be doing dishes today. Instruct them to use recyclable paper products unless they want to do the cleanup!

June 14

Needing a reminder is normal, and something to consider if you aren't able to remember to interrupt sedentary behavior. There are many studies that suggest sedentary lifestyle is more dangerous than behaviors such as smoking. So get up and move every hour, or better, every half hour.

It doesn't have to be exercise or even cause you to breathe heavy. Moving every hour is about becoming less sedentary, so anything goes. Simply standing up to greet someone or pacing while on the phone counts. If it's time for a break, you can work a bit harder and head up a flight of stairs for a bathroom break, or outside to take a jaunt around the block. Set your phone or other alarm to remind you to move. Alternately, some smart watches have reminder apps.

D.I.E.T. #166

Set a timer for movement, and when it goes off, don't ignore it! You don't have to stop working, but at a minimum, stand up for a moment.

June 15

There are a number of reasons for hydrating throughout the day, such as improving focus and controlling cravings. Oftentimes hunger is actually thirst in disguise, but eating snacks usually seems more satisfying than drinking fluids. If you are trying to lose weight or improve energy levels, consider the importance of hydration, as it is helpful in controlling portions at meals, which can improve control of blood sugar.

For the purpose of reducing calories at meals, drink water prior to eating. If this is done before every meal and snack, consumption should decrease, particularly if hydration has been a challenge for you. Aim to consume at least eight ounces of water prior to taking a bite. Of course, drinking fluids while eating is also recommended, to slow you down and increase early satiety.

D.I.E.T. #167

Drink water before every meal and snack. This is a simple experiment to carry out today. Take note of how it affects your food intake.

June 16

As a child, I don't recall thinking much about food. I think it was mostly because I was kept busy, and was blessed by a happy home. My mom cooked dinner most nights, and we would play outside at any possible chance. Being called in to eat was not something we looked forward to!

If childhood was not a happy time, think about how a happy child would feel about food versus playing. Most of them eat for hunger, and think about food when they need energy to play. While eating isn't necessarily torture to children, most kids could think of a million other things they'd rather be doing. Act like a kid today and find a childhood game to play, or call a friend for entertainment.

D.I.E.T. #168

Play like a kid again! While I loved to be around my friends, I also liked to go out and shoot hoops alone. It could last for hours! Today, find something you enjoyed as a child, and try it again.

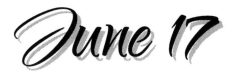

June 17

Take every meal outdoors today, even if it's hot or rainy. You might have to sit undercover, or in the car, but no matter the weather, make it a point to enjoy your meal outside of your normal quarters. Being out in the open air is helpful in improving attitude and becoming more mindful.

Switching up your environment is one thing, but getting Vitamin D from the sun and fresh air to breathe is the goal for mealtimes today. If you have time, go to a park and enjoy people watching, or head to an outdoor local concert where you can enjoy a sandwich and listen to music. If those locations aren't available to you, it's no big deal! Everyone has access to the great outdoors.

D.I.E.T. #169

Eat outside. Whether it's on your back patio, on a hike, or outside the office building, eat every meal while enjoying the summer season.

June 18

Most vegetables are considered "free" foods, meaning you can eat as many as your heart desires. The more, the better due to their dense nutritional content and low calorie nature. If only you wanted to eat endless amounts of vegetables, right? Consider preparing them in a big batch, in a delicious way.

Grills are great for steaks, but barbecuing foods other than meat is a great health goal. The grill allows starches to develop into sweet roasted flavor, and veggies become irresistible! My favorites for the BBQ include mushrooms, bell peppers, zucchini, cauliflower, asparagus, and tomatoes. Other hearty choices include onions, eggplant, and of course sweet corn.

D.I.E.T. #170

Grill vegetables today. Simply drizzle them with olive oil, and place in a grill basket or wrap in foil. Place over medium heat of the grill for four to ten minutes, depending on your choices, and turn once or twice until nicely browned and softened. Refrigerate leftovers, if there are any!

June 19

While daily cardio workouts are important, there are other things you can do to keep your body strong throughout the day. Using your core to function in activities of daily living will help prevent overuse of other muscle groups which often leads to pain and potential injury.

If something is to become a habit, it must be incorporated into your life in a simple way. One suggestion to improving core strength is to practice holding abdominal muscles tight while breathing. Find a time during the day that will provide you the opportunity to practice this exercise. A good example if you commute, or run errands daily, is to hold your abdominals in at stoplights.

D.I.E.T. #171

Find regular opportunities to activate core muscles. Decide now if it will be at stoplights, or if you will set a timer. Pull the belly in toward the spine, as if you were drawing in to zip a zipper. Hold that feeling, but continue breathing. Do this for as long as you can, or until the stoplight turns green.

June 20

Regularly perusing cooking magazines is a hobby of mine. I don't like keeping entire magazines, so I will tear out any recipe that meets my (and my family's) criteria for healthy and tasty. Though it requires review to avoid getting messy, these torn out recipes are placed in a file folder of "next to try" ideas. This simple folder gives me inspiration when having chicken again becomes an unbearable thought. After trial, each recipe makes its way into the binder of family favorites, or gets tossed.

Instead of agonizing over what's for dinner, make your own file and flip through the folder at the beginning of the week. If you don't have time to go grocery shopping, make sure you are cutting out recipes that use staple items you are likely to have on hand. Give some of your "next to try" ideas a shot. They might just make it into your collection of favorites.

D.I.E.T. #172

Start a file folder of new recipes to try, and revisit it weekly for inspiration and grocery planning.

June 21

Self-love is more important than any nutrition or exercise plan. If you don't care for yourself, your efforts won't last, and most certainly won't become habits. What does it mean to love yourself? It isn't about being arrogant, but about having positive inner conversations.

Unless you are very mindful and conscious of it, you probably don't know what you say to yourself throughout the day. However, every moment of the day your mind is thinking, creating judgments and opinions. A great way to change your thoughts is to start the day with a positive reflection. Tonight, use a sticky note to jot down one thing you are proud of. For example, consider what a best friend would say about you.

D.I.E.T. #173

Before you go to bed, place a self-love sticky note on a mirror where you will see yourself in the morning. This is a great exercise to repeat over and over, as you will reap long-term rewards for loving yourself more deeply.

June 22

Life is too short to be serious all of the time. Learning to lighten up can be hard for people who struggle with illness or who are trying to focus and stay on track. But realize there is a big difference between carelessness and being more carefree. In fact, it's helpful to loosen up the reigns, and you *can* do it without falling off course.

A step in the right direction is to laugh more. Find time to be silly, and if you have to, set aside five minutes to force a smile or two. Look up jokes or memes that will help you take the seriousness out of your day. Try to distance yourself from people who bring you down, and befriend those who make you laugh.

D.I.E.T. #174

Laugh today. Be silly, learn a joke, or read a meme today. While laughter burns calories, it also reduces stress through relaxation. Study after study have proven, happy people are healthier!

June 23

When there's not a lot of drama, there's also less need to seek comfort from food. However, if you have a lot going on, it is easier said than done to take emotions and circumstances away. In order to avoid coping with food, try to lower your emotional response to stress. How? By avoiding situations that you know are toxic, and by practicing relaxation techniques that help you blunt your response to stressful situations you can't avoid.

I love the quotes that remind us that we can't avoid rain, but we can dance through a storm. We can lower our response to storms in our lives by practicing how we act on our emotions. Breathe, take an extra second before responding, and be more in tune and thoughtful of your stress level.

D.I.E.T. #175

Eliminate unnecessary drama. Notice how you respond to stress today, and take an extra moment before eating to make sure it is for hunger.

June 24

Using a smart tracker to measure calorie burn is ultra popular, but there are better ways to measure success when working out. Torching five hundred calories is great, but what else does it do for your body? That is the real success. When burning calories is the focus, we begin to think that calories eaten can go up. It turns into a mind game.

Today's goal is to pick a new way to measure success. For example, if you are on a spin bike, the goal is to increase average cadence or resistance, which increases output. On a walk, try to improve the time it takes to walk a particular distance, which requires changing your pace. If you are lifting weights, the goal might be to perform one extra repetition of each exercise, which improves muscle endurance.

D.I.E.T. #176

Choose a new metric for measuring exercise success. If only for today, do NOT focus on calories burned, but on what other kind of step forward you can take in your physical activity.

June 25

Sometimes I get in a rut with eating because I get stuck on certain recipes and food combinations I like, and then find myself bored. For example, my favorite condiment is green salsa. On everything from eggs, to chicken, to avocados! However, I find that switching up sauces and flavorings is a great way to reduce boredom with healthy eating. Both green and red salsas are great toppings, but there are many others to help mix it up.

Look for a sauce or topping that won't add unhealthy amounts of sodium, sugar, and fat. It can be hard! At the very least, try to minimize your portion. An example is using different vinegars on veggies, or using hot sauce on eggs. Other less harmful condiments include Dijon mustard (and other mustards), pesto, and pickle relish.

D.I.E.T. #177

Use a flavor, sauce, or condiment that is different from your normal preference. When eating healthy gets boring, get creative!

June 26

Kindness is contagious, and it can certainly benefit more people than just the receiver. There are many ways to be kind, but the simplest way to include these random acts is to give compliments. Make sure your compliments are not just about appearance or material things. Notice another person's talent and tell them they are good at what they do.

Be genuine in your compliments. Seek out ways to encourage others by focusing on their strengths. You never know how much of a difference one simple comment could make to someone who is struggling, or to someone who needs one more little push. When you do this, there is a chain effect, and others down the line will also benefit. It can make a huge impact, and you will notice how this makes you feel more positive in your own life.

D.I.E.T. #178

Give at least one compliment every hour today. If you aren't around others every hour of the day, compliment yourself! Set a reminder to do this hourly.

June 27

The idea that chocolate is good for you is based on anti-oxidants. Oh, and it is good for you to consume things you really love to eat! To get more chocolate in your life, consider choosing a variety that provides the antioxidants with the least amount of sugar and fat. I'm talking about Cacao!

The cacao bean is where chocolate originates, and cacao powder is the bean, pressed and dried into a powder. The result is a dense source of magnesium, iron, and antioxidant-acting flavonoids. When ground into a powder, cacao makes an excellent substitute for traditional baking cocoa, and is a great way to turn smoothies into chocolate masterpieces!

D.I.E.T. #179

Use Cacao. It is widely available and easy to use. I use it so often that I devoted a canister to it, and have a scoop that makes it easy to add to my daily smoothie. Cacao also makes fantastically rich hot chocolate!

June 28

Most people are naturally goal oriented. Even if you aren't, making a list of things you need to accomplish is a great way to keep your attention set on your goals. Accomplishing items on the list can give you momentum to achieve the next thing! Here's what you need to do to get started TODAY:

- Record a short-term goal, or one you want to achieve in a month or less.

- Think about the events of the week ahead.

- Determine realistic mini-goals for this week that will help you reach your short-tem goal. Choose up to ten things to accomplish.

- Record at least one strategy that will help you achieve each mini goal.

D.I.E.T. #180

Here's an example: You might have a short-term goal of losing five pounds. Two mini goals could be logging your food intake and exercising daily. Strategies to achieve these mini goals may include taking your food journal to work and keeping your workout clothes in your car.

June 29

If you don't like to be noticed, today's DIET may be a bit challenging! What you wear can make a big impact on how you feel, so it's time to break out of a comfortable spot and wear something exciting, bold, or energetic. Then, let your appearance and how you present yourself guide your day!

If you normally wear dull colors, you might have to rummage through the closet, but it should be simple to put a pop of color on. Make it your goal to be "bright" today. It could be in the way you present yourself, or it could be in how you dress. One simple idea is to wear an accessory like a scarf, colorful bracelet, or watch. If you wear bright colors in general, try bright lipstick, or fun socks.

D.I.E.T. #181

Be bright. If this doesn't work for your wardrobe or makeup, have a bright attitude and choose brightly colored foods. Lighten your mood by wearing color today!

June 30

In the summer months, it's hard to stay cool and hydrated. It takes extra effort to consume enough fluids, even when you are thirstier. One simple step to keeping cool and increasing the amount of liquid you are taking in is to add ice to any smoothie, hot, or cold beverage.

It might seem obvious to add ice to a glass of water, but placing it in a larger glass so you have more room for ice will give you a colder, more hydrating option. Grind up ice in every smoothie you make, even if you have other frozen items in it. Instant hydration! Ice your hot drinks such as coffee and tea, as this also provides additional hydration. Even drinking a sports drink or recovery mix over ice will fill you up with healthy hydration.

D.I.E.T. #182

Use ice in everything you drink today. You'll feel better and more satisfied if you stay hydrated in the summer months. Cravings will be curbed and muscle cramps will be less likely.

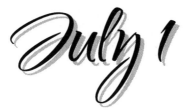

July 1

Exercise can be daunting when you have a specific task to complete, such as working out for thirty minutes or jogging three miles. Keeping it fun can be challenging. To mix it up a little, keep your workouts full of surprises by using dice to select your activities.

How do you use dice to workout? Assign specific activities to each side of the dice, or have someone else do it. Roll, and go! You can choose to do the number on the dice, such as one full pushup, or do a set number of a variety of exercises. For example, roll a one and you'll do ten pushups, or land a two and do ten jumping jacks. You could add treadmill time for rolling a three, or add rest time for rolling a six.

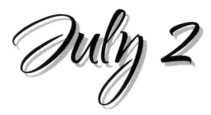

July 2

Goals are critical to any healthy journey, and setting mini, short, and long term goals is important. A stretch goal is one that you think is almost out of reach, or is out of reach at the present moment. The point of a stretch goal is to push you beyond what you think is possible.

Reaching daily or short-term goals is important to keeping momentum going. You've likely decided on a long-term objective, so think beyond that. It could be a reward for achieving that goal, such as celebrating with a vacation, or you could commit to another lofty ambition such as running a marathon.

D.I.E.T. #184

Stretch yourself. Striving for something you feel is out of reach is an amazing way to build confidence and feel accomplished. Remember that you likely don't know what you are capable of!

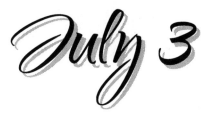

July 3

Smiling has the magical power of making you feel better, whether giving or receiving the smile. Even if it's been the worst day ever, smiling at people will improve moods all around you. Take a moment to notice the domino effect of genuinely smiling at strangers. Improving someone else's mood will improve yours too!

When you are happy, it is easier to make good choices. Even if you think eating isn't emotional for you, happiness can drive choices that are in line with your goals. For example, if healthy eating is your goal and you are feeling good, you will more likely make choices like skipping the drive through, prioritizing your workout, or avoiding afternoon caffeine.

D.I.E.T. #185

Smile at five strangers today. Not everyone will smile back at you, but maybe your kindness will be passed on to the next person they see. It's worth a try.

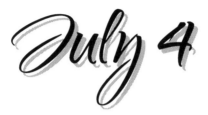

July 4

Watermelon is the first red food that comes to mind on a day like the 4th of July. It's a great summer food that most everyone enjoys. If you're trying to come up with a food to serve today, consider patriotic foods by the colors red white and blue, instead of traditional burgers and hot dogs. While it is fine to serve a meat item too, make your side dishes healthier than heavy pastas and Jell-O salad!

Here are a few color-coordinated ideas:

- Mozzarella, tomatoes and basil are a pretty appetizer. When placed on a skewer, they are perfect for a party!
- Strawberries and blueberries served with vanilla Greek yogurt are refreshing.
- Try blue corn chips with salsa and Cojita cheese for a snack.
- Serve angel food cake with raspberries and light whipped cream for dessert.

D.I.E.T. #186

Eat something red white and blue today. Instead of focusing on hot dogs and pasta salad, focus on serving and eating something with patriotic color.

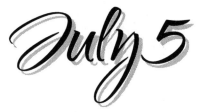

July 5

It can be hard to bounce back after a holiday, and it's easy to think, "I'll start next week." Start today! You can more easily incorporate a change when you don't overthink it.

Most of the time, it isn't the meal, but all of the extras that add up when celebrating a holiday. Don't stress out over yesterday, but be confident that eliminating these extras can help you bounce back. Today, skip the extras that come in between and after your meals. Desserts and sweets can be a big challenge, but cutting them out is totally worth it.

D.I.E.T. #187

Go back to your routine of having purposeful meals today and get rid of any lingering desserts. This will keep holiday sweets special, instead of turning them into a daily habit. Do it today and get right back on track!

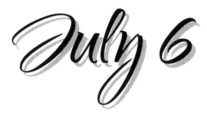

July 6

One of the best things about summer is fresh produce. It is plentiful and delicious, especially when July comes along. Farmer's markets are great places to find ripe, nutritious, local fruits and vegetables. Markets are typically limited to weekend hours, but farm stands might be able to fill in the gaps during the rest of the week. Getting your exercise walking around is an added bonus!

My favorite farm fresh items are tomatoes, cucumbers, greens for salads, asparagus, herbs, salsas, and ripe melons. There are plenty of novelties as well, so try to limit candies, breads, and dessert items! Once you've collected your bounty, take it home and clean it as soon as possible. Enjoy a salad with all of your ingredients, and savor the fresh tastes of summer.

D.I.E.T. #188

Go to a farmers market or visit a farm stand today. Have a plan in store for what you want to purchase, and what you want to prepare with your delicious finds!

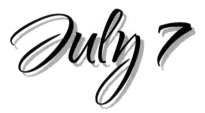

July 7

When was the last time someone gave you a compliment for a job well done? It feels good to get recognized for your efforts. Even if you haven't been encouraged lately, consider how much you praise others. Could you do more? Giving out praise will definitely help others, but it also feels good to know that you might be changing the world, one person at a time.

Giving a compliment is simple, but praise involves a bit more attention. Watch for a person who did something out of the ordinary, and then say something. It could be as simple as telling a young boy who held the door for you, "great manners, young man," as I have heard adults praise my son. Guess what, he keeps holding the door, in part because he was praised.

D.I.E.T. #189

Give praise. Yes, today is about treating someone else the way you want to be treated. It will come back to you, I can assure you of that.

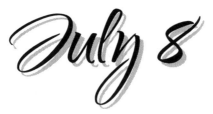

July 8

A toned flat six-pack of abs isn't achievable for the majority of people. It doesn't pay to focus on the appearance of one specific body area, but training the core for purposes of better movement, pain relief, or healing and preventing injury does pay off.

Strengthening the core muscles, including everything in the middle of your body, hips and low back, is something that takes persistence. Start it today, but make sure you are including a core activity most days of the week. Appropriate exercises involving the major core muscles include plank, lying leg lifts, "superman" style back extensions, and moving lunges. There are a million more, but these are some simple favorites.

D.I.E.T. #190

Work on your core. Spend at least five to ten minutes doing a variety of exercises, and repeat at least three to four times a week. You can choose to include core moves during regular exercise, or separately.

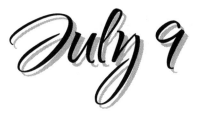

July 9

While suggesting to eat fresh, made at home meals every day of the week is what you might be striving for, you get a pass today on the fresh part. Trying to be perfect isn't the goal, but making habits that involve less eating out is realistic.

Using frozen items is one way to offer yourself a "pass," and it saves money too. Just because there isn't something defrosted doesn't mean you can't eat at home. Consider fish stick tacos, or whole grain toaster waffles with eggs and cheese on top. Do you have any frozen berries? How about smoothie bar for dinner, or using frozen cauliflower or broccoli to make a simple crust for pizza? Just steam, puree, add one egg, Parmesan, and some breadcrumbs.

D.I.E.T. #191

Head to your freezer for a meal. Take an inventory and get creative. You can find thousands of recipes on the web when you type in the ingredients you have on hand. Voilà!

July 10

Gardening, mowing, mulching, and yard cleanup is absolutely physical activity. When it's hot, I suggest adding watering to the list, so you can spray yourself to keep cool! If you make sure to slather on the sunscreen and drink lots of water, working outside will be one of the healthiest summer activities you do.

Not only is yard work calorie burning activity, it is strength building and can be relaxing as well, depending on what you are doing. The other benefit to working outside is that you tend to lose track of time and are distracted from mindless snacking that might happen if you were indoors! Collecting Vitamin D from the sun is another benefit, as the sun is the best way to absorb it aside from drinking fortified milk.

D.I.E.T. #192

Do yard work. Many people like to count it as a workout. Go ahead, yard work is hard work!

July 11

When you have to be a role model, eating healthy is easier. As a Registered Dietitian, eating well is my job, so I have it easy! To teach kids healthy habits, or to be a supportive spouse or friend to someone who is sick, you will likely eat better too. It's just what you do, because you care about others and want to show your support. You can take this approach in general, even if you don't have children or a sick loved one.

At lunchtime there might be others in your company and in your spare time there might be friends around you. Even if you are alone, act as an example for yourself! Do what you would do if there were someone around who needed your support, and you will be your own support too! Avoid heavy meals and sugary snacks, instead choosing fruits, veggies, and lean proteins.

D.I.E.T. #193

Be an example. Today, treat yourself the way you would treat another who needed your encouragement and wise choices.

July 12

There are many ways to make eating more natural. Peanut butter is an easy swap, now that many of the natural varieties have been made creamier and tastier. There is another way to improve it without buying it in a jar, and that is to grind your own. It really isn't that hard, especially if you have a good food processor.

It's as simple as dumping a handful of nuts or seeds into a processor or high-powered blender and pressing high. Alternate between high and low pulses until you have a butter consistency, about four to five minutes. Depending on the nuts you use, you may have to add a drizzle of oil to make it creamier. You can also roast nuts or seeds ahead of time to add toasty flavor. If you don't have a food processor, many grocery stores have nut butter grinders, where you can grind the desired amount into a container to take home.

D.I.E.T. #194

Grind your own nut butter. You'll not only reduce additives in your diet, you'll also enjoy a deliciously healthy treat!

July 13

Vegetables are a repeated D.I.E.T. for good reason. They should be a theme in our lives! It is definitely important to prioritize eating veggies, because they are easy to forget. To make it easy for today, plan to have them mid afternoon. Even if you don't typically snack, this is a good place to put them in, to increase your fiber intake and for added hydration.

If you tend to go overboard on your evening meal, vegetables in the afternoon can help fill you up and keep you from going back for seconds of your dinner. For a great source of fiber, try raw broccoli, carrots, or cauliflower with hummus. For a great crunch, go for snow peas or snap beans. Other ideas for additional fiber and hydration are bell peppers, celery, radishes, fresh mushrooms, and baby carrots.

D.I.E.T. #195

Snack on vegetables this afternoon. My favorite vegetable snack is cucumber slices with sliced cherry tomatoes and a drop of balsamic or rice vinegar.

July 14

Since it's my anniversary, I have to make D.I.E.T. 196 about celebrating. Every day should have a little special in it, because life is precious. So today, you are given the task to have a little fun. For some, this is a larger task than for others who may see every day as a party. Either way, let's get started!

Think about a time you achieved something. Did you celebrate? Did it include food or drinks? Likely! Today, celebrate your strength and perseverance using something other than food or drinks. Treat a walk around the block as a privilege, or appreciate a big glass of ice water for the refreshment it provides. Take the dog on a walk to celebrate you, or sit on your porch and soak up the sun in the peace and quiet.

D.I.E.T. #196

Celebrate yourself and your journey towards healthier. It doesn't have to be your anniversary to treat yourself a little special. And treating yourself better doesn't have to mean eating cake!
Make it a point to enjoy life today.

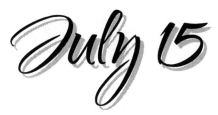

July 15

Eating more food in its natural form is a great goal, and today you can put it into practice by focusing on foods that don't have labels. This means you might swap eggs and fruit for breakfast and have a salad with grilled protein for lunch. Dinner would include meat and veggies, for example. There are a few caveats to no-labels eating.

Dairy products and soy protein foods have labels, as do frozen fruits and vegetables. These are fine to include, as they are naturally occurring foods that have been processed only in the sense that they have been packaged. Other processing such as removing the healthy part of a grain to make it white, or adding stabilizers and other hard to pronounce ingredients are what you should avoid today.

D.I.E.T. #197

Don't read any labels today. This means, don't eat any foods with labels! Except, of course the natural foods that happen to have labels on them.

July 16

Research shows that peak bone density in humans occurs at about thirty years of age, and slowly declines from there. Around menopause, bone loss accelerates for women, and these losses continue into older age for both men and women.

Eating enough of the right foods and performing weight bearing exercise will slow bone loss. Calcium and Vitamin D are the two minerals to look for. Calcium comes out of bones if there is not enough in the diet, and Vitamin D helps the body absorb calcium into the bones. So make sure you are getting plenty of BOTH! Dairy foods, salmon, sardines, dark green veggies, and almonds have a lot of calcium. Vitamin D can be found in dairy foods, egg yolks, and is plentiful from sunshine! Examples of weight bearing exercises include weight training, but also walking, jogging, stair climbing, or playing sports.

D.I.E.T. #198

Strengthen your bones today. Get outside to take a walk in the sunshine. Come in to a snack loaded with calcium and Vitamin D, such as a cold refreshing glass of milk!

July 17

Depending on what you eat, lunch can be the most important meal of the day. Having a small breakfast can help get your body started for the day and keep you going strong through the morning. If you limit your portions of carbohydrates and include some protein in the morning, you can make it through until lunchtime.

Eating half of your daily calories by the end of lunch is a reasonable goal. Doing this will provide the body with energy at the most useful time of day. Contrary to morning eating, having the largest meal in the evening encourages most bodies to store calories due to natural cycles of metabolism. For example, increases in insulin at evening mealtimes cause relative increases in fat storage.

D.I.E.T. #199

Make lunch your biggest meal. In order to provide the body with energy it can use throughout the afternoon, and in order to delay hunger at dinner, eat at least half of your daily calories in the first half of your day.

July 18

Instead of reading labels, counting grams, and adding up calories today, use your stomach to guide you. Thinking about hunger and fullness is an all day project. Most people don't eat according to hunger, but instead consistent to a schedule, or perhaps according to emotions. Today commit to listening to hunger cues that could include a growling stomach, empty stomach feeling, or slight dizziness.

Wait until you are 75% sure you can't wait anymore. What does *that* feel like? It means you start to notice physical symptoms, but are not weakened by them. You might get a slight headache at 75% or feel light headed, but you are not passing out or faint. You might have a bit less concentration, but you are not completely agitated. You might feel a gurgling stomach, but are not feeling nauseous.

D.I.E.T. #200

Think about percentages. Eat when you are 75% hungry. Wait a few minutes when you first feel hungry and see if the feeling passes. If not, make the choice to eat.

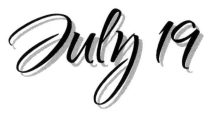

July 19

Hunger is your assignment again. Why two days in a row? Mindfulness is a process, and practicing it two different ways on successive days is a good way to see if it can help you meet your goals. Today, the strategy is different. Try to build on yesterday, eating when 75% hungry, but focus on only eating to a feeling of 75% full.

In this experiment, you'll decide what 75% full means to you! Typically, slowing down when eating can help a person feel fullness before getting to "stuffed." So, chew slower and notice when hunger starts to disappear. You might feel a slight pressure build in your stomach, which is a sign it is time to be done. Don't fret about food going to waste!

D.I.E.T. #201

Think about percentages again. Eat until you are 75% full. Remember, it is worth it to waste food if you can save your waist!

July 20

When food is considered a privilege, it becomes special and attention worthy. Many times, eating is taken for granted, and food is just something we need to get through the day. Truly enjoying it becomes a rare occasion, and enjoyment often times requires a bit of gluttony.

Instead of needing excessive fat, sugar and calories to enjoy a meal, pay attention to how much you can appreciate a simple lunch or snack. Crunching on a sweet apple and enjoying the hydration it provides can be an experience in mindfulness. Or, savoring the taste of a single bite is an experiment in how to get more of your senses involved in eating. Focus on moving food around in your mouth, noticing its texture, shape, and flavor for at least a few moments before swallowing.

D.I.E.T. #202

Today, don't take anything for granted. See the little things you have access to as blessings. Notice how this can affect what you choose to eat, and how you choose to eat it.

July 21

The treadmill and elliptical can be boring, and procrastinating exercise happens more often when these are the only means of getting moving. Structured exercise isn't as daunting as you might think, especially if you can find something you like to do. If you can determine a mode of exercise you enjoy, it will more easily become a lifelong habit.

Even if you are not an athlete, sports can be a great way to disguise a workout. It doesn't have to involve a team, but certainly could. Join a beginner tennis or golf league, or find a sand volleyball league. If competitive isn't your personality, take up speed walking or try a 5K training program. Rowing, swimming, and cycling are also great sports to play alone. Look for something accessible to you that could become a regular activity in your week.

D.I.E.T. #203

Play a sport today. It becomes more play than exercise when you can find activities to enjoy on a regular basis.

July 22

Variety is the spice of life, right? Trying to broaden your palate can be a challenge, and it starts at the grocery store. Purchasing and preparing new foods (or old favorites you forgot about) is a great goal for today. In order to include variety today, think about eating a variety of colors.

When selecting what to eat, look away from white foods and possibly even brown foods. Include bright colors like red, orange, yellow, green, blue, and purple. Eating all the colors of a rainbow at least once a day, or eating ONLY the colors of the rainbow all day long are two very measurable and achievable goals. It might be a challenge, but you will enjoy it more than focusing on what you *can't* have today.

D.I.E.T. #204

Eat the colors of the rainbow. Notice how your energy level improves by eating colorful foods. Take on the challenge of eating the rainbow of colors in foods. Blue and purple are the hardest, but you can do it!

July 23

It is helpful to experiment with different forms of exercise to avoid boredom in your routine. While it is summertime, aim to include more outdoor activities, so you can take advantage of the sunshine and warmer temperatures. If you like company, ask a friend or relative to join you to make the time go faster. Some dogs are great outdoor companions as well.

While walking or jogging can be enjoyable, hiking in a new area can provide a sense of peace that cannot be replicated when your route is through a neighborhood or on busy sidewalks. Drive somewhere to appreciate nature today.

D.I.E.T. #205

Take a hike today. It may not include a mountain or a field of tall grasses, but find a place you haven't explored before. Try to fully enjoy the scenery, breathe deeply, and appreciate nature. It will pay you great dividends, especially if you get a bit sweaty along the way.

July 24

I **used to purchase cream of this** and cream of that, corn bread mixes, spice blends, and buttermilk, among other random ingredients that a recipe might call for. Then I found it was cheaper and healthier to use the ingredients I had at home to prepare these things from scratch. It also saved time by preventing extra trips to the store.

You can do this too! For example, if you have a recipe that uses cream of chicken soup, try this: Mix ½ cup of milk with 2 ½ cups of chicken broth or stock in a saucepan and bring to a low boil. In a small bowl, whisk 1 cup of milk, ¾ cup flour, and ½ teaspoon each of onion powder, garlic powder, salt, and pepper. Pour the flour mix into the pan with the chicken broth mix and whisk over low heat to simmer. Continue to simmer about 5 minutes.

D.I.E.T. #206

Try a DIY version of an ingredient. Creating meals at home might mean using a few prepackaged items like canned beans and boxed pastas. However, many simple ingredients can be just as easy to make from scratch.

July 25

There are some foods that are worth the work of eliminating. If a food makes you feel sick, it seems obvious to avoid it, but if you feel constant fatigue or have bowel problems, this is also a time to take a look at the foods you are eating. See if you can make some connections between what you are eating and how you are feeling physically.

Try to identify a food that makes you feel less healthy, then make a commitment to avoid it today. It could be a food you know causes GI symptoms for you, one that is heavy in sugar and fat, or a food that makes you feel tired.

D.I.E.T. #207

Make food choices based on how you feel physically. If you know that a food causes bloating, avoid it today. If there is a food that gives you heartburn or makes you tired, skip it. It's only one day, but notice how much better you feel, then see if you can eat what makes your body feel good, more often.

July 26

Playing with dice to workout was something you may have tried already this year. Get those dice back out and use them for meal planning! Dice are especially helpful when you get bored, or are out of ideas for what to have for dinner.

Assign a protein to each number on the dice. Then, assign a veggie. Select a starch, dairy product, or easy side dishes for the rest of the numbers. Roll the dice two or three times to decide what you'll make. Recipes also work well for the game. For example, roll the dice once to decide on protein, then again to pick one of six recipes you have available for that protein. Kids love to get involved in this!

D.I.E.T. #208

Use dice to plan your meals today. Sometimes it works best on a day when you can get to the store, just in case you roll a number that requires an ingredient you don't have. Keep your dice and number assignments in a jar and get it out whenever you need meal planning help.

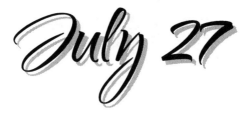

July 27

If you followed yesterday's challenge, you may have some ideas of what to pick up at the store! Having a variety of proteins and veggies on hand can be challenging enough, so focus today on taking an inventory of what you have and what you need. Creating a list can provide inspiration to cook at home, since you will have a plan of what to do with your groceries. It's easy to go shopping, but to go shopping with a plan and then follow through... now that is success!

You don't have to go to the store today, but make a list. Add to the list through the week, and go when you have more organized meal plans in place. Start your shopping with produce and proteins, then move to dairy, eggs and grains, plus ingredients for recipes. Here's the challenge: stick to your list!

D.I.E.T. #209

Make a grocery list. Keep it somewhere handy so you can add to it as you make plans for what you will eat this week.

July 28

Gluten free is a way of eating that most people have heard of. It is critical for people with celiac disease, but many others claim it helps with IBS, pain, and mood swings too. If you don't have celiac disease it isn't required, but it can be an interesting experiment to eat fewer carbohydrates over all, avoid obvious gluten, and see if you feel any different.

This style of eating is not very complicated for people without celiac. Avoiding obvious gluten means avoiding foods with wheat, barley, rye, and oats that are not labeled gluten free. You might think that means avoid carbohydrates, but it's not the same! You can have fruit, corn, potatoes, quinoa, beans, and rice, to name the most popular gluten free carbs. The main focus of gluten free diets for non-celiac patients is to eat foods that are naturally void of gluten such as lean proteins, fruits, and veggies.

D.I.E.T. #210

Go naturally gluten free today. If you don't have celiac disease, remember that gluten-containing carbs actually contain a lot of great nutrition, so eat them in moderation tomorrow!

July 29

It's a challenge to stay focused on your own individual goals. When one person is doing something that works, it is natural to want to try it too. It's also natural to have a bit of jealousy or desire for that same success. Social media worsens all of this, especially when a person is just starting out on a healthy journey.

While it is unlikely that social media posts are intended to make you jealous, it can happen. On the other hand, if you like to post your own success or photos, you may get upset watching who likes and doesn't like your post. To simplify your life today, see how it feels to completely ignore social media. At the least, you will enjoy your free time a bit differently!

D.I.E.T. #211

Designate today as a social media free day. Avoid posting, and avoid looking. Focus on you and your goals, work hard, and remember to be proud of yourself.

July 30

Today is an opportunity for a fresh start. In fact, at any moment, you can decide to push "reset" and start over. Purposefully doing what you need to do to restart is only possible when you *decide* to do it, and have a plan to follow. To reset your body nutritionally, you'll need to focus on hydration, fruits, veggies, and plant foods. Avoiding processed foods and sugar is also required, just for today.

For your fresh start, choose fruits for breakfast, beans and veggies for lunch (such as in a stew), nuts and fruit for snacks, and a giant salad for dinner (choose olive oil and vinegar if you want to add dressing). You can add a kale and fruit smoothie or extra veggies for snacks, and make sure to drink at least half your body weight in ounces of water today.

D.I.E.T. #212

"Cleanse" your body today by focusing on fruits, vegetables, beans, nuts and seeds for energy. Hydrate with water today. Notice how your focus and energy level improves!

July 31

Everyone has a "relationship" with food. It can only be made healthier by first realizing what kind of relationship you have. Do you avoid eating or forget about food sometimes? Or do you constantly think about food, worry about it, or hate how it makes you feel?

It is important to think about whether food controls you, and if you feel like you are constantly battling it. Food can sometimes be seen as the enemy, but once it is realized that food can't truly control anyone, a healthier relationship can develop. Whether you have a love for food, or feel like it's your enemy, find some relief by making peace. Decide that *you* are in control, because *you* are the only one who can truly make that decision.

D.I.E.T. #213

Make "peace" with food. Decide to be in charge of what you choose to eat, when you choose to eat it, and how much you choose to consume.

August 1

Sometimes tight muscles cause pain in joints or cause over-compensation in other areas. Almost everyone can think of a time where tight muscles kept them from exercising. Even if you aren't feeling tight today, focus on releasing a muscle group with a purposeful self-massage method.

There are many ways to loosen up muscle tissue. While a massage is lovely, it is not always accessible. Instead, use a foam roller, or perhaps more convenient, the edge of a countertop or tennis ball. Using a counter, lean into a muscle group such as the hips or back with gentle pressure. Lie on a tennis ball to roll over the back and glute muscles. Foam rollers work the best for legs and glutes. Spend at least five minutes per body part the first time, and give enough pressure to reach a slightly uncomfortable feeling.

D.I.E.T. #214

Try muscle release with a tool. Use something simple such as a ball or edge of a countertop, or consider purchasing a foam roller for future use.

August 2

When you are trying to make a change, there are challenging actions to take. Action steps are required when making lifestyle adjustments. Perhaps it would be advantageous to turn off the TV earlier or put on workout clothes when you get home. These are little decisions that, depending on your action, will either push you to achieve your goals or derail you. Even if you don't want to do them, you know that you should.

So how do you get over the lack of drive, or the stall in motivation? Don't think about it. Just do it without any hesitation. You may never want to put on your workout shoes over plopping on the couch, so stop waiting until you do. Don't pause, as you'll give yourself too much time to think. You'll put yourself at risk of avoiding what you need to do to achieve your goal. Instead, just get started!

D.I.E.T. #215

Don't pause with any decisions you know are important. Avoid overthinking.

August 3

There are many cooking methods that are healthy. Grilled or baked meals get the thumbs-up as low fat ways to prepare dinner. These methods are common, but not always simple, and certainly not always quick. There may be a lot of ingredients involved, or there may be a hot oven or grill to work around.

Steaming is another choice that retains nutrients, since it is a quick process done with minimal liquid. You can use the stovetop, microwave, or a steam or pressure based cooker such as an Instant Pot. Cooking foods by this quick method retains more nutrients versus boiling. Reusable or disposable steam bags can simplify the process for quick microwave steaming, no water or oil needed.

D.I.E.T. #216

Steam something. Try veggies in a basket on the stovetop, or in the microwave. If you've already mastered this, consider cooking a piece of salmon or chicken by steaming it in a pressure cooker. It's fast, easy, and healthy!

August 4

When the backs of your legs feel stiff, it is typically the hamstring muscles to blame. You may develop muscle imbalances and are at greater risk for pain and injury when you have tight leg muscles, since other muscles take over to help compensate.

If you loosen the hamstrings, you can move more freely throughout your day, and your risk for developing back pain is lower. If you have tight hamstrings and you already suffer from back pain, stretching them can improve your pain. A simple way to stretch: Sit with your back flat against a wall, sitting up tall and pulling the belly muscles in. Straighten your legs out in front of you. This might be challenge enough, but if it's not, bend forward from the waist, reaching the chest toward the thighs. If you prefer lying down, wrap a towel around the bottoms of your feet and stretch your legs straight upwards. You can also grasp behind one thigh at a time.

D.I.E.T. #217

Stretch your hamstrings. Hold stretches at least twenty seconds before resting and repeating three to five times.

August 5

Brainstorming is a great way to get creative with your goals. I recommend doing this with another person, to increase your ideas and expand your thoughts. Today, keep a pen and paper handy or use another device to record your inspirations.

Take at least ten minutes today, divided into at least two sessions, to think about what you want to accomplish the rest of this month and the rest of this year. Creating short term goals are the focus for today, and while most people know goal setting works, few of us actually take the time to think about how we can stretch ourselves. Brainstorming means writing everything down that you are thinking of, without judgment. Once you've spent three to four minutes writing, spend the last bit of time picking out two to three things to focus on in the short term.

D.I.E.T. #218

Brainstorm. It's amazing what can be discovered and developed when you allow your thoughts to spill out on paper.

August 6

Using recipes to make a fancy meal is fine when you have all of the ingredients. It isn't so great when you don't! Instead of relying on a recipe today, use the ingredients you have on hand. Picture this: you have chicken defrosted and leftover rice in the fridge, but not a lot of anything else. Here's a recipe to try using your basic ingredients.

Heat your oven to 400 degrees. Chop the chicken into pieces and place them in a baking dish. Top with a mixture of breadcrumbs, Parmesan cheese (optional), dried basil, pepper, and a drizzle of olive oil. Bake in the oven for 25 minutes, or until bubbly. Meanwhile, whisk 2/3 cup milk with 1 T flour and 2 teaspoons chicken bouillon in a saucepan, over medium heat. Cook until thickened. Add 1 teaspoon dried basil. Take your chicken out, serve it over rice with the cream sauce drizzled on top. Make a frozen green veggie to balance your meal. Voila!

D.I.E.T. #219

Make dinner without a recipe. It doesn't have to be chicken, but if you don't have a bunch of ingredients it doesn't mean you have to eat out!

August 7

If you've ever done an interval workout, you know it's a great way to get your blood pumping. Plus, you can get a post-workout high in a shorter period of time. You don't have to be in great shape to perform interval workouts, but you may have to modify the types of exercises you include. You should also make sure your doctor has cleared you for strenuous exercise.

High intensity interval training, or HIIT begins with a few minutes of warm up, followed by a period of work, such as twenty to thirty seconds. A recovery or rest period of ten to fifteen seconds follows the work. Repeat this work/rest pattern repeating one exercise, or a mix of several favorites. My favorite HIIT workouts combine cardio such as running or jumping rope with strength exercises such as pushups and squats.

D.I.E.T. #220

Do a HIIT workout today. Keep it simple by doing 15-20 rounds of work/rest using the same one or two exercises. Make sure your rest periods give you just enough time to catch your breath.

August 8

If you're exercising more and trying to eat right, you are likely trying to retain as much lean body weight as possible while losing body fat. It's not easy, but there are certain ways you can build your lean mass, and retain it while continuing to shrink additional fat stores.

One strategy is to consume plenty of protein, or at least half a gram per pound of body weight. More than that, up to .8 grams per pound is a guideline for muscle building/ strength training. Another important detail is to consume protein after workouts and at bedtime. Consuming dairy prior to bedtime can help in keeping lean muscle from breaking down while sleeping, and aids in building additional lean body stores.

D.I.E.T. #221

To add to your protein intake today with appropriate timing, choose dairy foods before bed. Milk, cheese, and yogurt are great examples of easy bedtime snacks. Dairy foods contain proteins necessary for building and retaining muscle.
Make sure you hydrate well when increasing your protein intake.

August 9

When things get tough, people give up. The human body was actually designed to protect itself from doing hard things, so it is almost as though we are wired to give up when faced with challenges that seem unattainable. Today, accept that you will have challenges and declare that you will see them through.

Remember the rainstorm analogy? Think about a child dancing in the rain. The child doesn't see the rain as threatening or annoying, or even as an obstacle to having fun. That's key! How can we return to our childhood roots and just dance through our rain? It isn't that simple, but be conscious today of what storm you might be facing, and how you can see it from a child's perspective. While it may never be fun, your rain will end, and you will be stronger having danced through it.

D.I.E.T. #222

Dance in your rain today. Whether it's a sun shower or a catastrophic storm, you will achieve greatness by learning to push through with a light heart and confident strength.

August 10

"**Ready, set, go**" is a phrase we learn as a child, and something we can return to as adults. It represents preparedness, confidence, and action. Similarly, counting "1, 2, 3" helps a person prepare to do something, recognize they will be taking action, and begin that action.

If you've ever seen kids jump into a pool together, they almost always holler ready, set, go, or 1, 2, 3. Why? To prepare, be confident in the action that is coming, and to carry out the action. Do they hesitate at 3? Sometimes, but you won't! Consider counting a helpful strategy in making decisions. When deciding whether to snack or not, consider counting 1, 2, 3, and then making your choice. This is a form of delaying your action. If you want to go for a run, you would count 1, 2, 3, and take off. Or choose to get up from the couch– 1, 2, 3!

D.I.E.T. #223

Count to 3. You'll take action if you give yourself a starting count, and it will eliminate the option of procrastinating.

August 11

Learning to eat a healthy diet is simple, but actually doing it is hard. If you've kept a food journal in the past, you might know that you don't eat enough vegetables, or that you aren't meeting your protein needs. It is okay to have a backup plan for catching any potentially excluded nutrients.

You don't do it on purpose. In fact, you may be missing out on nutrients because you are trying to reduce your calorie intake or your portion sizes. It's easy to do. It's equally as easy to pick up an over the counter multivitamin and take it every day. While not absolutely necessary, multivitamins can provide a safety net of nutrients that might not be consumed perfectly every day.

D.I.E.T. #224

Take your vitamin. Make it easier to remember by having a routine, such as taking it with other medications, or after brushing your teeth at night. It will be well worth the effort!

August 12

When you are distracted, it is easy to fall into mindless eating patterns. Eating by the television is one action that easily turns into a daily habit, and can decrease overall mindfulness. It can also create other problems, such as eating by the computer at work, or chowing down on appetizers while making dinner.

Attempting to incorporate mindful eating at every opportunity will be easier if you avoid distractions. Do that today by eating only with the television off. If you watch something at night, do it without eating. Avoid televisions if you are eating out, choosing to put your back to any screens. This strategy is best done for a few days in a row, to set a pattern in place that limits overall distractions.

D.I.E.T. #225

Avoid eating by the television. Sit while eating, but turn screens off, and focus on eating slowly and enjoying the taste of your food.

August 13

In the nutrition world, "SoFAS" stands for solid fats and added sugars. Reducing saturated or solid fats to less than ten percent of daily calories is a helpful rule, while limiting added sugars to less than ten percent of daily calories is also important to overall health. On a 2,000-calorie diet, these percentages equate to 22 grams of saturated fat and 48 grams of added sugar.

Remembering the SoFAS acronym can help remind you to limit these ingredients when shopping for groceries and when brainstorming snack and meal ideas. Aim to eat whole foods, and avoid packaged ingredients to help you meet the SoFAS goal. Examples of packaged foods that can still be included are cottage cheese, rice cakes, and salad mixes.

D.I.E.T. #226

Keep track of the SoFAS in your diet and plan to stay within the ten percent guidelines for saturated fats and added sugars.

August 14

Having a partner in your challenge to eat healthier makes it much more bearable, and definitely more maintainable. If you live alone, it is especially important to get outside support for your efforts. If you have family chaos, it is also critical to get buy-in from your relatives. Cooking with someone is one way to make it happen!

Decide on a menu and decide with whom you will be eating; then get to work! Enlist your helper in food prep, measuring, stirring, and/or plating and garnishing. Play music or have fun catching up on the day's activities. Share your reason for including your friend or family member, and make sure to include why you chose to ask for his/her help. Enjoy your company; then enjoy your meal together!

D.I.E.T. #227

Prepare a meal with a family member or friend. Focus on creating a vegetable and a protein first, then a starch or other side dish, if desired.

August 15

Opening your world to new flavors and combinations is a great way to get out of old patterns. If you always cook chicken the same way, it's not a meal you probably look forward to. Finding ways to make meals more interesting can keep you from heading out to eat and can increase your satisfaction from a healthy meal.

You can try a new ingredient, but better yet, cook a new food today. If you've never tried lentils or tempeh, these are great protein sources to rotate in. If you are interested in new vegetables, try a green such as broccolini, or a different type of lettuce like bok choy. Trying a likeable way of eating a new food such as cauliflower in crust or kale in a smoothie is another strategy.

D.I.E.T. #228

Cook a new food today. You may find a healthy favorite that provides variety to your meal rotations. If nothing else, you will gain a bit of an adventurous spirit!

August 16

Melatonin is widely known as a hormone your body produces to regulate sleep cycles. When secreted normally, it aids in your ability to fall asleep and stay asleep. Eating foods such as walnuts, oats, and bananas can increase melatonin levels, but there are other behaviors that will increase your body's ability to produce it's own sleepy hormone.

Blue light, such as that emitted from televisions or electronic devices, has been shown to reduce your body's production of melatonin. So, turning off those devices earlier can help you get sleepy faster. Give yourself at least thirty to sixty minutes of non-screen time prior to bed to help ease you into your own sleep naturally. At a minimum, avoid sleeping with a television on all night.

D.I.E.T. #229

Go to bed without any blue light. Spend time reading a book or magazine, taking a bath, or catching up with your spouse or kids. It's better quality time anyway!

August 17

Adding movement to every day is an important priority. It doesn't have to be extra time at the gym, and it could be as simple as changing the way you do certain things throughout your day. The recommendation of parking further away is a simple one, and the example of walking to speak to someone instead of texting them is another.

Using an elevator or escalator is faster, but taking the stairs is healthier. The three flights of stairs I have at work are not only calorie burners, but also energy boosters. If I have to catch my breath, it means I did something that woke up my metabolism. Seeing it as energizing instead of exhausting can keep you motivated to do it day after day.

D.I.E.T. #230

Take the stairs today. Eventually, you'll look forward to trips up the stairs at work, and you'll find yourself looking for other opportunities to slip extra heart pumping activities into the day.

August 18

Chronic dieters welcome the chance to avoid reading labels! Even if you are simply monitoring overall nutrition, taking a break from all of the numbers and using a more abstract method is healthy for your mind! You'll likely want to continue this method versus tracking and counting everything you consume. The good news is that it works better than all of that counting, because you are eating what your body needs in a less stressful way.

Aim for balanced eating today by dividing your plate into fourths. One fourth should contain starch, one fourth can be protein based, one fourth should be fruits, and the last is veggies. Dairy on the side or extra veggies counts as a bonus. Alternately, dairy can be considered your protein. This helps in the case of breakfast, if you choose to have Greek yogurt instead of eggs or sausage!

D.I.E.T. #231

Use a plate to visualize your meals divided up into the kinds of calories you need. Focus on portions and attempt to build healthy variety into your meals.

August 19

While barbecues in the summertime are popular, you don't have to limit yourself to a grill. Light up a campfire or a fire pit and get cooking! You may think of this type of cooking as only for hot dogs and s'mores, but today, get creative and cook a healthy meal over an open flame. Try a fire pit or campfire, or very carefully, use a gas flame.

Kebobs work well for an entrée item, and they limit charring of items due to reduced time over the fire. Take care to avoid burning your food, as the compounds that form during that process have been shown to be harmful to your overall health. Get your veggies in by roasting them over the fire. Some of the best veggies for this method of cooking include bell peppers, onions, summer squashes, corn on the cob and hearty mushrooms. You can even grill lettuce such as hearts of Romaine!

D.I.E.T. #232

Cook a food over an open flame. Don't limit yourself to s'mores! Kebobs, red peppers, corn on the cob, and hearty mushrooms work great and are full of nutrients.

August 20

Avoiding added sugar has been a strategy in many previous D.I.E.T.S. Being more specific about how to do this can be helpful. For example, eliminate any added sugar in the beverages you drink today. Added sugar can be found on the ingredient list as many titles including: brown sugar, corn sweetener, corn syrup, dextrose, fructose, fruit juice concentrates, glucose, high-fructose corn syrup, honey, invert sugar, agave, maltose, malt syrup, molasses, raw sugar, sucrose, sugar, syrup, and others.

Sugar comes in many forms, and many so called "healthy" drinks include lots of added sugar. Reading an ingredient label is the best way to eliminate these added sugar sources. Milk and 100% fruit juice have natural sugars, which are fine to consume in proper portions. Even better, stick to drinks that don't have labels, such as water or coffee.

D.I.E.T. #233

Eliminate sugar-sweetened drinks today. And of course, take care to avoid adding sugar yourself. This includes honey, syrups, agave, brown sugar and table sugar.

August 21

A great way to improve your calorie intake is to share meals. My parents do this, and since it's their anniversary, it's a great strategy to share! In addition to encouraging each other to make a healthy choice, you'll also help your sharing partner develop a habit of proper portion control.

This strategy can work while eating out, as well as when cooking at home. Eating half of your usual quantity will greatly reduce your calorie intake. Having smaller portions still allows you to enjoy something delicious, but also helps you realize that the portions served are typically more than you need.

D.I.E.T. #234

Share a meal with someone you love. Help each other be healthier by choosing a moderate meal and cutting it in half. You'll notice that sharing still allows you to fill up, and that you don't need the huge portions that you might be used to eating.

August 22

Physically and mentally putting an end to something is helpful in changing habits. Simply "trying" to eat better or exercise more is likely not enough to convince you to continue making the right choices day after day. Making a commitment to something in a bigger way is important. Taking a physical action to mentally commit might take some creativity.

To make a bigger impact on changing your habit, try something such as releasing a balloon or burning a habit written on paper. If you're near an ocean, a message in a biodegradable container is fun and memorable. Flushing something written on toilet paper is also silly but actionable! Be strong about your intentions to be healthy. Take remarkable actions that state, "I am done with you, bad habit!"

D.I.E.T. #235

Say goodbye to a bad habit. It doesn't matter how, but do something to physically and mentally be rid of it.

August 23

Most people admit that they don't eat enough vegetables. It can be hard to consume enough unless you focus on it, since starch and protein usually get most of the attention. For example, steak and potatoes are protein and starch, but a lot of people might add a dinner roll on the side. Choose salad or steamed spinach instead! Plan to have two different vegetables at your evening meal, or choose to have double portions of your veggie.

Strategizing is important when setting a goal like increasing vegetable intake. Keeping frozen items on hand, chopping and prepping ahead, visiting farmers markets, and having salad items available are all helpful. Having a plan in mind for how to use your produce will assure that it gets consumed before it goes bad!

D.I.E.T. #236

Eat double vegetables at dinner. Do this by having seconds of your veggie, or serve two different choices. Focus on non-starchy options such as greens, squash, tomatoes, broccoli, mushrooms and peppers.

August 24

My grandfather was best known by his grandkids as a fisherman, and he loved nothing more than to take his family out to the lake, catch some fish, and camp a few nights. We loved to watch him catch a fish and clean it, and then watch my grandmother cook it for us to eat. There is something about seeing the process of sea (or farm) to table that turns food into something more than just tasty grub.

You will know what I'm talking about if you have had the privilege of catching fish, or farming crops and creating meals out of your efforts. The satisfaction from these types of meals is unmatched! If you don't have access to fishing or farming, growing tomatoes or herbs in a pot is another way to enjoy garden-fresh ingredients.

D.I.E.T. #237

Eat something from the sea, unless you don't have access. As a second option, choose a farmed crop. If you don't have access to crops, plan to pot an edible plant or a tree that bears fruit.

August 25

It's true that giving is much more satisfying than receiving, and it doesn't have to cost anything. Giving supportive advice, a helping hand, or a listening ear can be better than any gift you could buy. It will offer you fulfillment, and giving can help you feel needed and appreciated.

Today, think of a friend who may need cheering up. You could choose a coworker that seems down in the dumps, or your neighbor who always seems to be helping you. Consider providing fresh cut herbs or an extra tomato from your farmer's market bounty. Or, make a homemade salad dressing and pour it into a cute glass jar. Tie it up with a ribbon and write the recipe on the outside.

D.I.E.T. #238

Thank a friend with a healthy treat. Don't bake desserts or provide a gift of wine this time. Instead, try to give away some of what you are learning on your own healthy journey.

August 26

If you are trying to make a big difference in your dietary intake, or in the overall quality of what you eat, give up something that will provide a major impact. Eating meals from drive through restaurants not only packs in calories, but also provides little nutrition for those calories.

It's definitely easier to have someone else prepare your food, but it doesn't have to be. Just prepare a few things ahead of time. Toast a waffle on your way out the door, hard boil eggs, prepack nuts and cheese, purchase fresh fruit, and chop veggies. You'll be able to pack a meal together in no time. Whether it's breakfast, lunch, and dinner, or just an afternoon coffee, skipping the drive through today will encourage the beginning of a much better pattern.

D.I.E.T. #239

Avoid the drive through. Swapping out a fast food meal for something packed at home can save you hundreds of calories and offer you tons of extra nutrients. You'll enjoy a meal that can slim you down instead of weigh you down.

August 27

Often times, eating mindlessly happens because of lack of directions. When given instruction, most people can follow a list or stick to a plan. However, don't feel like you have to listen to someone else recommend things for you. You know your body best!

Design your own plan by creating rules that are realistic, achievable, and helpful to you as an *individual*. A helpful part of this strategy is creating lists that offer options for when you feel like snacking. Create a list of "go-to" foods you will keep on hand. These should include a crunchy veggie, a sweet fruit, a portable nut, and a filling dairy product. It could be more complicated, such as veggies with hummus or yogurt with berries, or it can be simple one-item choices.

D.I.E.T. #240

Make a "go-to" list. Go to the grocery store and fill your cart with your items. When hungry, insist on choosing only the foods on your list. If you can't choose one of them, you are most likely eating for reasons other than hunger, and should reconsider.

August 28

Sometimes good intentions to eat at home result in munching while preparing a healthy meal. Let's face it, cooking involves some prep work, and you might be feeling hungry, even if you're just bored or stressed! You need some distraction while cooking, so instead of turning on the news or having a glass of wine, turn on the music.

Music is a wonderful mood booster and can be a distraction from physical hunger. Turn on something energizing, or listen to a playlist of your favorites. Make sure it is a genre of music that makes you happy, and potentially invites dancing while you cook! Make a plan for what you will listen to now, and plan to avoid eating before your meal is on the table. Note: tasting foods for seasoning is excused!

D.I.E.T. #241

Listen to music while you cook. If you're going to do something while you prepare your meal, dance instead of munch!

August 29

When you hear "eat more whole grains" you might think of switching out your sandwich bread to wheat. This is one way to do it, but today, get more creative with including whole grain in your diet. Any grain in its whole form can be included. I suggest corn, oats, rice, and quinoa as easy options. Here's how to make sure you are doing it right:

First, check your ingredient label to ensure the word "whole" is included with the grain. You could choose brown rice cakes, popcorn, or oat bars, but it's even better to eat your grains as purely as possible. Some simple examples are steaming brown rice with your dinner, or upgrading to nutrient dense quinoa. You'll notice extra satiety and longer lasting energy from including portion controlled whole grains in your daily diet.

D.I.E.T. #242

Eat a new whole grain. The benefits are numerous, including the addition of fiber, protein, B vitamins and minerals such as magnesium.

August 30

The most important part of getting something done is avoiding procrastination. Have a sense of urgency. Just do it! Take this approach with groceries. Don't wait until you need to prep a meal to portion your groceries. Part of putting your groceries away should be making them useful. For example, when purchasing bulk items such as nuts, put them away in one-ounce containers instead of keeping them in a giant bag.

Portion snack items such as crackers and chips for lunches, and place them in a drawer or cabinet for meals to go. Divide up as many items as possible and package them as you would if you were taking them with you for the day. This also works well with produce to assure that it gets eaten, and with sweets, to assure you eat small portions!

D.I.E.T. #243

Divide groceries into portions when you put them away. If you do it right away, you'll thank yourself later.

August 31

In all my years of practice, the most universally successful approach in coaching behavior change has been to educate. To explain how the body works and WHY something needs to change helps people take the plunge and get started.

Whether your journey is just beginning, or is something you've been doing for years, there is always something new to learn. When you learn about what is going on inside your body, and what behavior change might do to improve your situation, you are more likely to give up old habits and be willing to change. For example, when someone understands what diabetes means and how treatment strategies work, they are more likely to buy healthy foods and eat at home more often.

D.I.E.T. #244

Learn something new today. Purchase a book by a credible author, listen to a podcast, or sign up for a class taught by a clinician. If you go online for information, make sure the website is medical, or at least science-based.

September 1

There's a lot to be said for taking a moment to interrupt your usual pattern. For example, instead of immediately snapping back at a coworker, take a moment to breathe and change your usual tone of voice. Take a moment to interrupt your usual pattern of honking at a stoplight and you might change the course of someone's day.

Waiting to decide how you are feeling before choosing to eat more is a strategy to reduce overeating. Get up and fill your water glass, or wash your dinner plate off. Decide if you are still physically hungry. Put a time limit on your break, spending at least three minutes doing something other than eating, before you decide to fill up again.

D.I.E.T. #245

Wait 3 minutes before having seconds. Watch the clock and be controlled about it. Relax and enjoy conversation, or think about what you are going to do after the meal. If you continue to feel hungry after your time is up, serve yourself an additional small portion.

September 2

Spicing things up can slow down eating, make it more enjoyable, and some studies show it can even speed up metabolism. Some people don't tolerate spicy foods as well as others, and certain levels of spice can exacerbate conditions like heartburn, stomach ulcers, and ulcerative colitis. However, most people can endure at least a bit of added heat.

For beginners, adding flavors such as green salsas, chipotle peppers in adobo sauce, or green tobasco can be tolerable and can slow down consumption of meals such as egg dishes, meats, and of course Mexican cuisine. When given a choice, ordering foods with a bit of extra heat is another way to control portions of ethnic foods such as Thai or Chinese cuisine.

D.I.E.T. #246

Add hot sauce, spicy salsa, or jalapenos to at least one meal today. Try chopping peppers to add a very small amount of spice, or use mild versions of salsas and hot sauces.

September 3

When junk food is out of sight, it might be easier to avoid. On the other hand, accessibility to healthy options is also helpful in improving your eating habits. Maybe not so easy, but organizing a healthy snack area can encourage consumption of healthy foods by making them easily accessible.

Select a spot for your snacks, either in the refrigerator or in the pantry, or both. If you don't want to have a whole drawer devoted to it, place a container inside of a drawer to go to. Fill your snack area with cleaned fruits and veggies and dairy items like cheese and yogurt. In the pantry, choose single serve items or foods that have been portioned ahead of time, such as snack packs of whole grain crackers or nuts.

D.I.E.T. #247

Make or organize a healthy snack drawer. Switch your focus to your approved "go-to" snacks in your healthy area, and you'll train your mind to forget about the junk food!

September 4

Achieving success might feel undeserved or uncomfortable. Maybe you don't like to hear people say, "Wow, you've lost weight" or "what are you doing lately?" These comments can make you think about how things were when you didn't prioritize your health so much. It might be tempting to slip into old habits. Do something to make your new habits more permanent, or to prevent yourself from giving into temptation.

If you have old clothes that are now too big, you might feel bad about buying new ones, but don't! Throw your clothes out, so you won't be tempted to fit into them again. Today, clean out your drawers and your closet. You might save one pair of jeans or a top, just so you can remind yourself of your success. The key is to only look at them for motivation and not to save them for when you need a pair of "fat" pants.

D.I.E.T. #248

Throw out clothes that are too big. Get rid of the possibility of ever fitting into them again!

September 5

Discovering a new snack that helps satisfy a craving or slow down your munchies can help when you are establishing healthy routines. A more exciting snack can save you from giving up on a routine that is boring and lacks variety.

Eating fruit as a snack is healthy, but can definitely be uninteresting. Make it more fun to eat by freezing it! Choose easily frozen fruits such as berries, grapes, or slice up bananas and freeze for slower consumption. You can add nut butters to banana slices, or freeze avocado chunks for smoothies. Choose a fruit to freeze today, and enjoy the endless possibilities of a more interesting snack item.

D.I.E.T. #249

Choose freezer safe containers or bags, and enjoy the longer shelf life of a frozen fruit snack!

September 6

It can be hard to understand our true ability, until we achieve something we once considered unlikely. Challenge yourself, or have someone else challenge you today. There are many fitness tests you can try to test your strength, endurance, and will!

Try a timed leg exercise first, such as a wall squat. Holding a static position such as this serves as a great test for muscular endurance. Standing against a wall, walk your feet away from the wall. Slide your back down the wall, bending at the knees and continuing to walk feet away until your thighs are parallel to the floor and knees are at a ninety degree angle. Make sure your knees remain above the ankles, not poking forward. Maintain centered knees, so that toes point straight ahead and knees do not sway in or outward. Hold this wall squat for as long as possible.

D.I.E.T. #250

Hold a wall sit for as long as possible. Record the date and your time, so you can improve as you get stronger in your exercise routines.

September 7

Leading by example is one of the most important trials of parenthood. Being a healthy example is easier for me when I include my kids in more of the food and activity decisions. If this is a challenge for your family, modeling a healthy life for your kids can start simple, with lunch making.

Provide a template for your kids, and follow it yourself too! Teach what a dairy product is, then offer choices. Offer various protein choices such as hard boiled eggs and steamed edamame versus sandwich meats only. Create a menu of sides such as baked crackers, fruit, veggies and hummus, nuts (if allowed at your school), and filling favorites like pumpkin seeds or popcorn. Require a fruit or veggie choice, and a hydrating, non-sugary beverage.

D.I.E.T. #251

Make your lunch with your kids' lunches. Use the template: protein source, dairy product, side, fruit or veggie and drink. Lead a healthy lifestyle and be an example with a home-packed lunch!

September 8

It is proven that lowering stress is critical in improving the function of your body, and/or in allowing weight loss to happen. In particular, noticing if you have anxiety around mealtime or when you are hungry is important so you can improve how you respond to it.

Consider that a bit of hunger is not a crisis, and in general, it is not something to worry about. Allowing yourself to be hungry, then breathing and realizing that you will survive is a very effective method to weight loss. It increases the time between feelings and reactions, and helps a person realize how much control is actually possible.

D.I.E.T. #252

Go hungry. Pay attention to feelings of hunger, physical or emotional, and wait them out. If you never feel hungry today, that is something else to consider. Challenge yourself to at least one hunger moment that you sit through and manage without food.

September 9

Measuring what you consume and improving it is usually more helpful than attempting to consume what someone else says is ideal for you. This is especially true with hydration, because there are so many lofty suggestions as to how much a body needs. Many times these goals are twice what a person is currently consuming.

Track what you consume now, and if it is less than 64 ounces, aim to increase your current intake by eight ounces per day, until you get to 64. Decide when you will drink the extra cup, ideally not before bedtime. Try to achieve eight-glasses per day. If you are overweight or active, increase it slowly, to as much as half your body weight in ounces of water.

D.I.E.T. #253

Track your water intake today, without judgment, and without altering your normal routine. Find out how far you are from your goal, and increase daily until you reach it!

September 10

If you live alone, it can seem like a lot of work to cook for yourself. Remember, you are worth it! Cooking a few portions of single serve meals can work for individuals, couples, and for busy families. Making double batches is a great technique for families who eat at different times of the evening, and making half recipes is helpful for single people. Freezing extras is a great way to always have something healthy, quick, and tasty on hand.

Single serve items can be made from entrée style meal items like meatloaf or egg casserole, by using a muffin tin and forming "muffins." Meatballs or baked chicken can also be portioned easily. Cooking a main meal such as eggplant Parmesan or chicken enchiladas can be done on a weekend and portioned into freezer size containers for lunches or for dinner later in the week.

D.I.E.T. #254

Make a single serving meal today. You can make multiple servings to freeze for yourself or serve a late dinner guest.

September 11

Human interaction is a psychological need, and connecting with people is a core part of being emotionally healthy. When we interact in positive ways with others, it feels good, and it builds our inner soul. No matter how sensitive or expressive we are, or are not, there is a benefit to connecting.

Physically connecting by hugging is one way to interact, and while not everyone loves a giant bear hug, there is benefit to offering one! Don't wait for someone to be sad to give hugs. Offer them to your kids, family members, and neighbors. If you have pets, hugging furry friends can offer great returns too. There's a reason why there is a type of therapy that involves hugging sessions!

D.I.E.T. #255

Hug at least five people today. Don't save hugs only for grieving, but do consider how you might change someone's day with a hug. You might also make your own day, since you'll likely feel great about your interactions.

September 12

Deep breathing, or belly breathing is a great way to relax, but it can also help relieve pain and make you more mindful in general. You have to try it to believe it, so here's how.

Lie on your back with your knees bent and feet flat on the floor. Place your hands on your belly, right over the navel. Notice whether your abdomen moves up and down with your breath. Now, inhale through your nose a bit longer, until your belly moves upward. Exhale through your mouth slowly, as long as it took to inhale. Feel your hands lower with your breath. Continue this pattern, aiming to move the belly with the breath, and matching the length of your inhales with the length of your exhales.

D.I.E.T. #256

Learn how to breathe with your belly. While you can do it sitting up, lie on your back when you are learning how. Notice how it makes you feel later in the day, and try it again whenever you feel stressed, anxious, or hungry.

September 13

When trying to improve habits, it is helpful to be able to avoid temptations all together. While it is important to learn how to better cope with temptation you can make it easier on yourself by removing the problem for a while. If it's a favorite food, you may be able to reintroduce it in controlled portions later, but for now, don't keep it in the house.

Desensitize yourself to a food that may be too hard to resist at this point. It's hard to avoid temptation when it's right there in your kitchen! So, make it easier on yourself and throw it away! There is likely something in your kitchen today that is making your journey more difficult than it needs to be. If it's a homemade goody that you feel bad about eliminating, give it away!

D.I.E.T. #257

Throw away one trigger food. If you feel guilty about wasting, remember, you might feel equally as guilty indulging in it over and over.

September 14

Measuring portions is helpful, but measuring them and packaging them up for later is smart meal prep. The more prepared you are, the easier it is to eat healthy, and the more habitual it will become. To be more accurate, use measuring cups or a food scale to portion out snacks or side items. Place them in plain sight where they are quick and easy to access.

Read labels or utilize a reputable website to determine what a 100 calorie portion would be. You might be surprised at the volume of almonds you will get versus the volume of popcorn! When you measure foods and package them up, it makes it a bit more scientific. You also train yourself to slow down and plan instead of just ravage the cabinets.

D.I.E.T. #258

Make 100-calorie packs for your fridge and for your cabinet. Decide which snack items will be on "standby," ready to be consumed when you have a snack attack.

September 15

Purchasing a variety of fresh produce is a great way to keep healthy eating interesting, but sometimes produce doesn't last as long as you'd like. To improve shelf life, certain fruits and veggies should be refrigerated, and others should sit alone on the counter. What about those bananas that all turn brown at the same time?

If you're like me, there may even be bananas on your counter right now. Everyone sees them, but there's usually at least a couple that get too brown. Peel them, slice or cut in half, freeze, and enjoy them in a quick smoothie. A serving size for a banana is one half, so the proper portion can be made ready in your freezer!

D.I.E.T. #259

Freeze bananas for smoothies. Use a frozen half of banana, one half cup of your favorite milk, and one half cup of your choice yogurt. If you need extra protein, add a scoop of protein powder, or use a Greek variety of yogurt.

September 16

There are many ways to increase the fluids you drink during the day. Some people don't have a problem hydrating, but for those who don't love to gulp water all day long, using a reusable straw might help.

The recommendation for water intake remains a minimum of 64 ounces per day, but that is often not enough. If you are active, more muscular, or trying to lose weight, you may need up to half of your body weight in ounces of water, each day. I recommend starting with half of your desired weight if you are heavier than you'd like. To encourage sipping all day long, try using straws today. Use a bigger straw to get more, and a reusable straw is my preference! If you have a reusable straw, put it in a large tumbler glass and refill until you reach your water goal.

D.I.E.T. #260

Use straws today. See if it encourages sipping more, or if you drink faster and easier. Some people swear by this technique, while others think it slows their intake. Test it out and see for yourself!

September 17

This journey is all about you, but turning your attention to someone else is important in your own success. The feeling of cheering for another person is quite different from the feeling you get as the person being encouraged. Urging a friend or a stranger to keep going can inspire you to challenge yourself to higher goals, and can remind you of how important you are to others.

When I used to run races, I admired the people on the sides of the road with signs and bells, screaming for the people running by. They were encouraging perfect strangers. Then I took part in this, from their side, and saw how it feels to help people who are working to achieve difficult goals. Take a turn today cheering for someone, no matter what challenge they are facing.

D.I.E.T. #261

Cheer for someone else. Whether it's a football game, race, or even an emotional issue, cheering someone on is contagious!

September 18

Prioritizing self-care can be difficult due to time constraints, finances, and overall lack of attention. Picking one treatment to prioritize is a simple way to give yourself the time you deserve to relax and rejuvenate. If you aren't one to have others care for you, schedule a time when you can do it yourself.

Especially in the fall, dry weather begins to set in which causes skin and hair to dry out. Picking a treatment that will benefit you with moisture could be a great choice. Try a deep conditioning treatment for hair, or purchase a packet of a deep conditioner and complete this at home. A massage is another great thing to prioritize. To DIY, some of the benefits of massage can be achieved with a foam roller or a tennis ball.

D.I.E.T. #262

Schedule a massage, hair, or nail treatment. You can schedule it at a salon, or plan a time to do it yourself at home.

September 19

Entertaining doesn't have to go away when you are trying to be healthy. In fact, it is a great challenge to try and stay on track when socializing. Share your goals with others, or keep them to yourself. Some people will embrace your goals, while others might do the opposite. Try to invite those who are positive, but if you don't have such a selection of friends, keep this challenge to yourself. It might be harder, but you'll feel empowered by your self-control!

Try planning a progressive dinner, or a potluck style meal. Ask guests to bring a healthier version of their favorite dish, or keep it less obvious and assign courses such as salad, green vegetables, and a whole grain. If you are planning to do it all, have a calorie free beverage available, and provide your own healthy appetizer such as veggies and hummus or mini cucumber sandwiches.

D.I.E.T. #263

Plan a progressive dinner or potluck with friends or family, for the purpose of challenging yourself in a social situation. Make staying on track a priority, but don't feel obligated to tell others.

September 20

Making eating an occasion is a practice that can enhance your satisfaction and reduce eating that happens due to boredom and emotions. Using a special dish or china, or getting out your fancy silverware can slow you down and make you think a little more about the experience of eating.

Why does eating out seem so enticing? Beyond the food, it is likely a change of environment and the idea of a different atmosphere. So, why not take that to your own kitchen? It could be a serving dish, but consider your utensils and eating dishes too. Set the stage for a different eating experience, as if you were celebrating a special occasion. See how this mindset affects the rate of chewing, conversation you might have, and amount of food you consume.

D.I.E.T. #264

Use a fancy dish or your treasured china. You deserve a special eating experience, and you can have one in your own kitchen!

September 21

Reflecting and adjusting is important whether things are going well or not. Being honest with your progress and challenging yourself to achieve more can keep you motivated and move you to higher goals you may not have realized were possible.

Take a few minutes today to remember how far you've come. Flip back to a few previous D.I.E.T.S. or look back at your journals. Remember advancements in your fitness, new foods you've tried, changed habits, and possibly weight or size that you lost. Take note of your anxiety or stress level and consider how it has changed. Then, write down your next set of goals, based on all you have accomplished.

D.I.E.T. #265

Reflect on your year so far. Today is a checkpoint, as there are 100 challenges remaining this year. So evaluate and congratulate yourself, or if you need to, adjust and hit the reset button.

September 22

Why do people participate in "spring" cleaning? Is it that motivation is higher in the spring? Maybe it gets them ready for summer? Consider doing a little "fall" cleaning today, to motivate you to be in your kitchen more. It is not inviting to cook at home when there are fingerprints and crumbs everywhere, so work on improving that and you'll want to spend more time preparing healthy meals and snacks.

Start by deciding on appliances you use often, such as the toaster and microwave. Wipe them out, clean out trays, and shine exteriors. Then move on to the stovetop or oven. I suggest using a self-cleaning cycle if you have one and if the weather is warm enough to leave the windows open. If not, wipe exteriors and clean up spills. Finish by shining countertops.

D.I.E.T. #266

Spruce up your kitchen by wiping crumbs and polishing appliances. You'll more likely want to cook at home if your environment is clean and shiny, and you'll feel a sense of accomplishment doing it yourself!

September 23

Even though the number of restaurants near you may be different than the number near me, there are likely at least a few to choose from within a bit of a driving distance. Open your mind a bit today and consider checking out a restaurant you haven't tried before, or choose one with healthier selections.

Many salad focused spots and "vegan" or ethnic restaurants are popping up, especially as eating trends become healthier. Be adventurous and try a place you may have avoided in the past. Order plant based meals, grilled options, and/or vegetable and whole grain based entrees. One of my favorite places serves quinoa and lentil burgers, and mac and cheese made with mushrooms and cashews (a vegan's dream!)

D.I.E.T. #267

Explore a healthier restaurant today that you haven't visited before. You might just find a new favorite. If nothing else, you will expand your palate and your willingness to try new flavors.

September 24

"**If you can't say something nice**, don't say anything at all!" Remember that this rule applies to how we talk to ourselves too. The amount of silent talk we participate in is incredible, and many more thoughts are kept to ourselves than are said out loud. The impact of those thoughts is greater than we realize.

Send your mind more positive messages, and train yourself to talk more sweetly. One method to learn this habit is to speak kindly to yourself while looking in a mirror. You've likely heard of this strategy and shrugged it off, thinking it is weird, useless, or conceited. However, start this quick routine and you'll notice how it changes your thoughts all day long. Do it for days on end, and you will change how you see yourself.

D.I.E.T. #268

Speak kindly to yourself in a mirror. Focus on your character, such as, "I am strong, and I am worthy" or "I am honorable, and I am trustworthy."

September 25

Caffeine is a tough habit to break. It can become an addiction when physical symptoms set in, but it is usually a habit well before it becomes an addiction.

Whether it is used for physical or mental reasons, avoiding caffeine for a day can help you feel empowered. It is achievable and measurable, and this goal is certainly helpful in improving focus and energy in the long run. Break the streak of coffee shop stops and save your cash for something else. Avoid the morning cup of coffee with a quick workout instead, and skip the afternoon soda machine by walking a few stairs during your break. Adding a kick to your heart rate by getting active for a few minutes will make you forget about the need for caffeine.

D.I.E.T. #269

Avoid caffeine today. Get natural energy boosts from water and decaffeinated beverages and use activity to jolt you out of an afternoon slump.

September 26

Plant based diets show a lot of promise in their ability to reduce risk for disease. The vegetarian way of eating excludes animal proteins, and might also exclude their milk and eggs. It can, however, include tremendous amounts of fiber, nutrients, and an appropriate amount of protein. In addition to the health benefits, vegetarians enjoy eating in a way that is friendlier to animals and the environment.

If you want to try vegetarian for a day or longer, focus on including proteins such as beans, lentils, and soy at every meal. Add nuts and seeds, choose whole grains instead of white or enriched versions, and enjoy fruits and vegetables often. If you want to include milk and eggs, you can boost your protein intake even more, and try vegetarianism in a bit milder fashion.

D.I.E.T. #270

Eat vegetarian today. If you decide you want some animal products, include milk and eggs, as a lacto-ovo vegetarian.

September 27

Meditation doesn't have to be complicated or intimidating. Deep breathing, practicing mindfulness, and prayer are all ways to calm the mind and stave off anxiety. To do it in a more purposeful way today, find a place to sit quietly. Then follow these steps:

Sit up tall, without resting against anything. It can help your balance to cross your legs in front of you, but if this isn't accessible, lying down is another method. If you are lying down, bend your knees and place your feet flat on the floor. Imagine your spine stacked in alignment and your hips directly underneath the spine (if you are sitting up). Close your eyes and deepen your breathing. See the darkness behind your eyelids and notice the peace of your body. Disregard pain or ill feelings. This is the hardest part. Just continue to breathe.

D.I.E.T. #271

Meditate today. As a person with chronic pain and anxiety, I can attest to the calming nature of meditation.

September 28

Taking a break from work, extra activities, volunteering, and other time consuming endeavors can provide time to rejuvenate and reset your motivation. Reducing stress and increasing enjoyment will provide a multitude of benefits to your journey.

This doesn't mean taking a break from being healthy with your eating and activity, but the intention is to remove yourself from your usual patterns to give your mind a break. Try challenging yourself with a day off, or plan a mini weekend away. Say no to additional activities, or plan a weekend or evening of nothing to do.

D.I.E.T. #272

Take a break. Cut yourself some slack by removing extra work and commitments. Keep your commitment to eating healthy and exercising, but take everything else off of your plate!

September 29

There are many ways to improve your protein intake. Protein has a variety of functions in the body. In general, it can increase lean tissue and help people eat smaller portions, which can decrease the amount of body fat they have. In addition, protein can help stabilize blood sugar and can reduce soreness when taken after exercise. Most active people need about half a gram of protein per pound of body weight. You may want to track your intake for a day to determine if you are eating enough.

If you need more protein, it's easy to add with a supplement. While I like to suggest high quality protein foods, you can also obtain high quality protein from whey or egg white protein powders. If you wish to try a vegan variety, brown rice, pea, hemp, and others are easy to find. Mix protein powders with a liquid such as water or milk of your choice. You can also try adding them to oatmeal, smoothies, and baked goods.

D.I.E.T. #273

Try a protein supplement. One serving is typically one ounce, but check the label to make sure.

September 30

It is a good idea to physically and mentally take a break to eat. The habit of eating "on the run" and the idea of multitasking during mealtime can become problematic when it comes to your health. When our minds are crowded with too many tasks, we tend to eat too much, and it's easy to neglect food quality. This can also lead to eating another meal often without a hunger cue.

Focusing on eating and enjoying can help you become healthier in multiple ways, including reaching your healthiest weight and improving your mental health around food. It can be made easier with one simple step. Put yourself in a physical position to allow focus. The best way is seated, without distraction, to help you recognize flavors, fullness, and satisfaction.

D.I.E.T. #274

Sit down every time you eat, even if it's a small snack. This will discourage mindless grazing, and encourage eating off of dishware instead of out of packages. Most importantly, it will give you the experience of respecting and enjoying the food you are eating.

October 1

When the weather starts to cool off, especially in the evenings, it is nice to enjoy a warm dinner at home. While a comfort meal of meatloaf and mashed potatoes is tempting, think about a meal that can be prepared quickly, or in advance, and still provide warmth and satisfaction.

Stews are simple and versatile, and can utilize a variety of ingredients you already have on hand. Pick a starch, a protein, and vegetables. Choose corn, potatoes, noodles or rice for your starch. Add a protein such as lean stew meat, diced chicken, lentils, beans, or shrimp. Then, choose your veggies. Tomatoes work well, as do celery, onions, peas, and carrots.

D.I.E.T. #275

Make stew today. Use a bit of broth to create the liquid, then dump all ingredients into a slow cooker and let it go! If you like the stovetop method, make sure you cook your starches and meats ahead, then combine with liquid and veggies, and simmer for 20-30 minutes.

October 2

Following basic etiquette rules can put you in the moment and force you to be more aware of your food intake. Mom always said to sit up straight, and for good reason! It helps to bring thought to how full you might be getting and how tight your pants might feel. There are other manners that can help keep you from stuffing yourself silly.

For example, before you start eating, take a moment to place a napkin in your lap. This breaks up any patterns of hogging down your meal as soon as you are seated. Take a moment to look at your plate, appreciate your food, and slowly begin. Then, keep your elbows off the table while eating! This behavior is another one that improves posture and helps you be more aware of how much you are consuming.

D.I.E.T. #276

Put your napkin in your lap and keep your elbows off the table! Especially if you eat alone, eating with manners will help you slow down, be satisfied more quickly, and respect your fullness.

October 3

Produce is better in quality and taste when it is in season. While a farmers' market bounty is great in June, there are many seasonal options in the cooler months too. There's something more delicious about certain foods and ingredients in the fall months, and I'm not just talking about pumpkin pie! For example, I really love apples in the fall. There is nothing like picking them yourself, but if you don't have access to an orchard, even grocery store apples are much better in their peak season.

Once you have your favorite apple on hand, stick it in the fridge for a little extra crunch and refreshment. Look forward to your snack, and notice the taste of the apple as you take your first bite. Appreciate the crunch, the sweet, and the juiciness as you work your way to the core.

D.I.E.T. #277

Enjoy the simplicity of a crisp apple from the fridge. There is nothing like a crunchy apple in the fall to keep you on a healthy path!

October 4

It is easier to accomplish a fitness goal taking one step at a time. It's why D.I.E.T.S. 365 was created! Today, this can mean taking one movement at a time. Start by choosing to focus on your upper or lower body. Then, select a movement that incorporates many muscles of the upper or lower body. My favorites are pushups for the upper body or squats for the lower.

Once you've chosen an exercise, make sure you know proper form; then make a plan for getting it done! I suggest completing 45 seconds of work followed by fifteen seconds of rest, repeated two to three times. Plan to do this at least three times today.

D.I.E.T. #278

Focus on a single strength movement in your exercise today. You should certainly add cardio to your day, but first make sure you can accomplish your chosen movement at least three times today.

October 5

If you don't have a plan for dinner yet, today's strategy can help. Eating leftovers is a great way to stay home and eat food that you already paid for and spent time preparing. Leftovers are certainly beneficial for your budget! If you eat them for at least one meal today, consider the money you saved.

It costs nothing to eat leftovers, and it saves time and energy as well. It also allows you another healthy home cooked meal, if that is what you have on hand! Choose leftovers from your fridge for lunch if you already have dinner plans. If you don't have anything to choose, plan to make extra for dinner tonight. That way, you'll have some for tomorrow!

D.I.E.T. #279

Eat leftovers. It's a great way to save money and use up perishable items. It also keeps you from the temptation of making a less healthy choice when eating out.

October 6

Everyone benefits from relaxation, but when you are anxious, angry, or sad, it is especially important. However, when emotions are high, it can be challenging to get to a point of relaxing. Use a purposeful action such as taking a "time out." You can go back to your issue after your time away, and you'll most likely have a better way of managing the situation.

Do this today, whether you have a truly stressful moment or not. It could be just a break from your routine. Take your time out by moving out of your current environment and focusing on your breathing, relaxing your muscles and maybe stretching. Do your best to eliminate any thoughts, continuing to shuttle them away if they come back during your time out.

D.I.E.T. #280

Take a time out. Do it with purpose, physically removing yourself from your environment if possible, and taking a few minutes to breathe calmly and send your thoughts away.

October 7

Mama always said breakfast is the most important meal of the day. Today, take it a step further. Make breakfast at home. This seems obvious to those who can't get going without a little fuel, but a majority of people still skip it, or eat breakfast with the help of a drive through.

It can be calming and refreshing to sit down to a meal in the morning. Since you will need to plan to get up at least ten minutes earlier to accomplish this, you may have to follow through on this D.I.E.T. tomorrow. You can create a make-ahead breakfast tonight to speed up the morning, such as by soaking equal portions of oats, yogurt, and milk in the fridge. These "overnight oats" can be customized in the morning by topping with nuts, dried fruits, and flavorings such as cinnamon or vanilla extract.

D.I.E.T. #281

Eat breakfast at home. For those who don't want to plan to cook an egg, try overnight oats as a simple and satisfying breakfast.

October 8

Learning is key to being motivated to change. Knowing how your body works, recognizing risk factors you have, or how a chronic disease can harm you makes your health a more urgent priority. Even if you don't have a disease now, today's D.I.E.T. requires looking up a health topic that applies to you in some way.

Maybe there is a history of heart disease in your family. Even a distant relative with high cholesterol is enough to warrant some research. Search reputable organizations for information, such as the American Heart Association, American Diabetes Association, or the American Cancer Society, depending on your interest. Make sure you read about the disease itself, and how you might be at risk. Some cancers, heart conditions, and diabetes are certainly inherited, but there are also a lot of preventative measures you can explore. Knowledge is power!

D.I.E.T. #282

Learn about a disease. Search management and prevention strategies, and decide which actions you are willing to take to manage and/or prevent disease.

October 9

A messy refrigerator can be an obstacle to efficiency in the kitchen. It can be a recipe for distraction and can hold tempting foods and condiments until you have a moment of weakness. On the other hand, a clean refrigerator can help you feel organized, motivated, and in control!

To organize your fridge, remove all items, but be prepared to move quickly, to prevent spoilage. Remove shelves and containers and clean them with soap and water, or another food safe cleaning solution. Diluted vinegar works well and is a natural disinfectant. Check all expiration dates and wipe down lids, jars, and undersides of milk cartons and other messy items. Replace your food strategically, choosing to discard of items that distract you from your goals.

D.I.E.T. #283

Clean the refrigerator. Start inside by removing food and wiping down shelves. It's a great way to clear out outdated foods and take inventory. After you've finished, make a list of grocery items to replace or add to your fridge.

October 10

Unfinished water bottles are one of life's greatest annoyances! When entertaining, there are typically at least a handful of bottles left on the counter to dump and recycle. It's an example of something we can all work on... finishing what we start!

Filling washable, reusable cups and bottles is a great environmental practice, but if you happen to drink from bottles that are not washable, at least make them reusable. Refill and drink from used water bottles again. Pay attention to how many bottles you might be using on a regular basis, and determine if you can reduce that number. If you don't use them normally, be mindful instead of what you are leaving in your cup. Finishing the last few sips, every time, can add to your hydration.

D.I.E.T. #284

Finish what you start. Finishing your water is a great start, but this concept can certainly be applied to other projects you have going today.

October 11

There are many types of squash to enjoy this time of year! Winter squash are harvested in the fall, and can be enjoyed throughout the winter. They have a very long shelf life, especially when compared to summer varieties, which makes them a great staple to purchase in the fall months.

Nutritionally speaking, squash provides low calories for its nutrients. Winter varieties are typically rich in fiber, B Vitamins, potassium, and Vitamin C, and have thicker rinds, allowing their shelf life to be much longer. Examples include spaghetti, butternut, acorn, and delicata squash. Summer squash grows fast in the summertime, and is best enjoyed quickly due to its shorter shelf life. Common summer varieties are zucchini, yellow crookneck squash, and patty pan.

D.I.E.T. #285

Harvest, or purchase a winter squash. Enjoy a home-grown acorn squash or purchase one at the store. You won't have to use it right away, but make a plan such as spaghetti squash Parmesan, or roasted butternut squash soup!

October 12

For me, buying groceries without taking inventory typically ends in extra bottles of vinegar and more chicken in my freezer than I need. Many people buy groceries without a real plan for how they will use them. This eventually results in waste and in eating out.

It is very likely that you have more food available in your home than you are aware of. Take an inventory today and see how many days of meals you could make without going to the store. You may have to purchase eggs, milk, and a few other perishables, but utilize as many frozen and pantry staple items as possible.

D.I.E.T. #286

Plan as many meals as possible from the groceries you have in your house right now. You might have to get creative, but challenge yourself to at least one week of meals without a major grocery trip.

October 13

One of the biggest influences on mindless or unintentional eating is advertising. It is easy to be unaware of it, but marketing can change our cravings and makes us eat for reasons other than hunger. There is a reason why restaurants run television ads near meal times! It is hard to avoid all marketing, but try and eliminate some of the exposure you get to food ads by limiting your viewing of commercials.

Now that shows can be watched ad-free, or at least on demand, recording and watching shows later is a great strategy to lessen the influence commercials can have on our eating habits. Even if you don't think so, the subconscious mind is noticing the bubbles of soda and steaming hot pizza, even when you aren't hungry! Today, limit your viewing of commercials by watching TV only when you can avoid or forward through them.

D.I.E.T. #287

Don't watch live television today, to limit the influence of marketing on your food choices.

October 14

Emotions can have a great impact on eating, both positively and negatively. When anger is harbored, or resentment is kept inside, it causes a lot of stress that can result in eating for reasons other than hunger. Practicing forgiveness and understanding is a great way to release the emotion, and gain some freedom from emotional eating.

Whether it is for something small, or for a major problem, forgiving an unkind word or action can be harder than it seems. Telling the person that you forgive is a major step. Writing a note, or repeating the forgiveness out loud also helps. While some things are never forgotten, prayer and meditation can help clear the mind of the unkind action or word. Remember that forgiving can provide freedom from your own suffering, and can certainly help you make better food choices.

D.I.E.T. #288

Forgive someone today. Even if only slightly, it will relieve you, and help you have freedom from potential emotional eating.

October 15

Quick cooking is made easier with kitchen gadgets and appliances such as the microwave. Not all microwave cooking is off limits. There are certain foods that turn out delicious and can retain their nutrients, contrary to popular belief!

All cooking processes cause some loss of nutrients to the cooking liquid, and heating foods changes the chemistry, no matter what method you use. Let's remember that eating vegetables that have been prepared in a microwave is better than not eating them at all! Steaming is my favorite method for cooking veggies, and this can be done with a reusable steam bag placed in the microwave. No water is necessary, and any liquids that come off are easy to pour back into the bowl after cooking.

D.I.E.T. #289

Use the microwave to cook vegetables. Steam bags are easy and quick, but you can also steam in a glass dish with minimal to no liquid added. Expand your options to include microwave cooking, so you can enjoy a quick veggie tonight!

October 16

As the season turns more "brisk" in temperature, it is the perfect time to think about brisk exercise! What exactly does this mean? Most people think of fast, but brisk actually refers to the intensity level of exercise. Finding a brisk pace requires walking in a way that increases your breath and raises your heart rate into an appropriate training zone. For most people, this means you can talk to a person next to you, but not in full sentences.

Feeling a bit breathless may be uncomfortable to you, but if you are in good health, it is critical to keeping your heart and body healthy. Today, challenge the intensity of your exercise, and see how fast you need to go to raise your heart rate and become slightly breathless. You can choose to increase intensity by adding incline or speed, carrying small weights, or by using better body mechanics such as good posture.

D.I.E.T. #290

Find a "brisk" walking pace. Then challenge yourself daily to find this brisk pace.

October 17

When a low sodium diet is suggested, most people think it means flavorless. But, it doesn't mean you can't have *any* salt, and it also doesn't mean your diet will be boring! There are many salt substitutes and other ways to improve taste without adding sodium.

Salt is the number one source of sodium, and if you can eliminate adding it to your food, you will likely meet a "no added salt" diet restriction. However, when a person has high blood pressure, heart disease, or family history, salt may need to be more carefully considered. Reading labels and restricting sodium to less than 2,300 mg is the American Heart Association's general guideline. Choosing low sodium foods and lots of produce, along with dairy products can improve blood pressure. Trying a salt substitute is a great way to improve the flavor of low sodium foods.

D.I.E.T. #291

Experiment with low sodium flavor enhancers. You can use salt substitutes, salt free seasonings, or herbs and condiments such as parsley, basil, garlic, lemon juice, vinegars and mustards.

October 18

If you've followed this book in order, you've read about setting alarms to get up and move, or setting an alarm early to enjoy the sunrise. Today, work on your hydration by setting an alarm to drink water. Even if you are drinking other fluids during the day, remind yourself to drink water on purpose.

Determine how much you need to drink, and how often, then set your reminders to drink. For example, if you need to drink 72 ounces of water in a day and you drink eight ounces with each of three meals, you will need to find time to drink 48 more ounces (24 ounces plus 48 equals a daily total of 72 ounces). You could set six alarms, two hours apart, and drink eight ounces for every alarm. If an alarm falls near a mealtime, drink both your mealtime water and your alarm water.

D.I.E.T. #292

Set alarms for drinking water. It may seem overly structured, but notice how it makes you feel compared to your regular hydration habits.

October 19

Including specific produce items in your day is a very direct and achievable goal. However, counting your servings is another way to include enough fruits and vegetables without being so picky about the types. It is important to have produce accessible at all times, but it can be challenging to keep fresh greens and perishable items on hand.

Aim for three servings of fruit and three servings of vegetables today. You can include starchy or non-starchy veggies, and can include the higher sugar fruits like bananas. Of course, if you have greens and non-starchy veggies or berries and melons available, these have more nutrients per calorie. The goal, however, is to count and achieve the recommended servings.

D.I.E.T. #293

Count your fruit and vegetable servings. A medium piece, half a banana, or one cup sliced fruit qualifies as one serving. One veggie is typically two cups greens, one cup non-starchy such as cucumber or tomato, or a half-cup serving of starchy veggies such as potatoes and corn.

October 20

Sometimes waiting is the hardest part! It's exciting to be in the spirit of Halloween and of all of the fall holidays coming up. The spirit, however, does not have to revolve around food and the traditional sugar and calories of the season. Feel free to purchase costumes, décor, and other fun holiday items, but avoid shopping for seasonal foods until the very last minute. Even then, you could likely avoid the sugar and fat by giving away coins, pencils, stickers, and other goodies.

Candy isn't off limits all together, but for today, commit to waiting until the last minute to buy it. Purchase other items, if desired. A sweet smelling holiday candle is an example of something that can get you in the mood without adding dense calories to your day.

D.I.E.T. #294

Wait until the last minute to buy Halloween candy and other seasonal treats. Today's strategy is specific—avoid the candy aisle!

October 21

Some people use photos to document their progress, while others use them to drive motivation. I'm not a big advocate for posting photographs for others to see, but posting them for your own eyes can be a helpful practice. Place them in spots such as the kitchen snack cupboard or in your car's cup holder, so you can remind yourself to make choices that are in line with your goals.

Regardless of whether your photos are from when you were larger, or when you were smaller, or just from when you were younger and had more energy, they can serve to remind you that working hard is worth it. Remember that skinny doesn't equal happy *or* healthy, but weight loss can equal better energy levels, a sense of control, strength, and a better overall quality of life.

D.I.E.T. #295

Look at old pictures of yourself, and decide if they would help keep you motivated. If so, post them in strategic spots to remind you of your life journey.

October 22

Snacking on high quality protein foods can seem boring and more challenging than reaching for something higher in sugar, carbohydrate or fat. It can be time consuming to cook proteins, and it can be expensive too. Something easy and relatively inexpensive for its nutritional value is a hard-boiled egg.

The perfect hard cooked egg is easy to peel, and shelf stable for a few days. Poke a small hole in the large end of your eggs with a safety pin, then place them hole side up in a steam basket. Add a bit of water to a pot on the stove, then cover and steam for about ten to twelve minutes. After steaming, place eggs in ice water until cooled. Tap the end with the hole on a hard surface, roll the egg around gently, and run under cold water to peel.

D.I.E.T. #296

Hard boil eggs. With the method above, you will be able to easily peel the eggs under cold running water.

October 23

Getting up in the morning is a chore for most people. There are some who spring out of bed, but many others who need to hit a snooze button or ask for a reminder. Whether it is physically hard to get out of bed or you just want to put off the workday, getting up in the morning takes a bit of momentum. There are, however, many experts who say that the most successful people in the world are those who get up and go to bed early.

Delaying the beginning of your day only sucks more energy from you. While it's hard in the moment, it is worth the effort every time. Remember to be grateful, stretch, and rise with a positive attitude. It will change the direction of your day!

D.I.E.T. #297

Don't hit the snooze button. Get your day going, spend a few extra moments relaxing, and you'll get to avoid the rushing around that happens when you snooze.

October 24

There are a few times a year when it gets harder to prioritize healthy eating and exercise. Around the holidays, there are extra stresses, and there are cooler, shorter days that might prevent you from getting outside. Since it is doubly hard to stay motivated, take today to write down what you will accomplish by the end of the year.

Two months is not very long, and this time of year is typically full of additional activities and gatherings. So, consider what you can realistically accomplish. Create at least one goal that is food related and one goal that is fitness or wellness related. Then, develop a list of small steps that will get you to the goal. An example is avoiding weight gain during the last two months of the year. Small steps might be to save sweets only for gatherings, and to avoid eating out unless for a holiday related gathering.

D.I.E.T. #298

Start an end of the year goal sheet. You have a couple of months, so make sure your goals are challenging, yet realistic.

October 25

An inviting work environment can improve motivation. In the kitchen, tidy countertops and shiny sinks are healthier and they are more fun to be around! Get motivated to cook in the kitchen by doing this one small step today. It might involve more work if you have lots of clutter or dishes in the sink, but it will improve your efficiency in the long run.

Today, clean your counters. Start with clutter. Clear off everything from your counter, placing it on another surface. Sort through mail, discard items that have been collecting, and put away anything else that has "landed" on the counter. Next, wipe down your counters and do your dishes. Use soap and water, or food safe antibacterial cleaner, and shine the sink. Now you're ready to food prep!

D.I.E.T. #299

Clean your countertops. It's motivating and healthy, and it could improve your mood if you are a clutter queen (or king!).

October 26

Lighting a candle is a great way to relax and enjoy a nice scent throughout your home. Just as simple is to fill a pot with water, bring to a boil, and add your own natural ingredients! Whatever you are in the mood to smell can likely be cooked up in your kitchen.

You may have heard them called "simmer pots" but call them what you will... the smells of fall are what matter to me on a crisp October evening. Some common simmer pot recipes include boiling apple peels, orange peels, cinnamon sticks, bay leaves, cloves, anise pods, pine, rosemary, lemon, vanilla, and nutmeg. You can leave them simmering on low all day, but be sure to add water as needed, as the liquid will evaporate. Refrigerate the leftovers if you like. They can be kept and reused for up to a week.

D.I.E.T. #300

Boil a source of natural fragrance. Fill your kitchen with amazing scents of the season!

October 27

It is the time of year when people start talking about holiday meals. It can be fun to come up with something new, but sometimes changing it up results in something not so great! Instead of experimenting, ask for recipe favorites from a friend or relative. Or, suggest a healthy holidays potluck at work. Participants can bring recipes for the healthy items they contribute.

Not everyone is a great cook or wants to make something homemade for a potluck. However, there is more than likely someone close to you who can lend you a hand with your task today. Be prepared with a healthy recipe of your own, holiday related or otherwise. A good place to start is a side dish, as the main course is typically easier to plan. A recipe such as a whole grain based side, green veggie, or a fresh salad with a great dressing is a fair and healthy option.

D.I.E.T. #301

Trade a recipe with someone. Ask your coworkers, neighbors, friends or family for a new idea. Then share your own favorite healthy recipe with them.

October 28

Pumpkins are all over the place! Now that it is close to Halloween, carve yours up and save the seeds. These tasty little morsels are packed with fiber, protein, and magnesium, and are a great source of potassium too. To enjoy them fresh, scrape them out of your pumpkin, soak them to remove the pumpkin pulp, and dry well on a paper towel lined baking sheet.

When they are dry, remove paper towels, toss seeds with olive oil and seasonings of your choice, and spread in a single layer on your baking sheet. Roast at 325 degrees for 20 to 30 minutes, stirring at least once. Cool, season again if you like, then enjoy! Store in an airtight container at room temperature, or in the refrigerator if you need them to last longer.

D.I.E.T. #302

Roast pumpkin seeds, or buy them already done. Store-bought roasted pumpkin seeds or "pepitas" are a deliciously quick and healthy snack. A proper serving size is about one fourth cup.

October 29

Fall is the perfect season for soup, especially as the temps start to drop. Pack extra nutrition by using colorful ingredients for the base, adding protein rich extras, and vegetables to increase fiber and fullness. One example is butternut squash soup with white beans added, or tomato and lentil soup with spinach or kale added.

To make a soup such as this, a simple online search will lend you a recipe. If you wish to create it on your own, start by cooking the veggies you wish to include, with seasonings as desired. Garlic and other fresh herbs such as rosemary, basil, and ginger are yummy in soups! Add dried beans if you are using them, or cooked proteins such as rotisserie chicken. Fill with broth, and let simmer to cook beans, warm proteins, and mingle flavors. Additional veggies such as greens can be added toward the end.

D.I.E.T. #303

Make soup! Get out your favorite recipe or create it yourself, and warm up a cool night.

October 30

Even though the selection may be less, waiting until today to purchase candy was smart! You likely avoided eating excess sweets because you limited your access. Now, purchase one bag of something you would not normally choose. If you like chocolate, go for the fruity candies, and if you like fruity flavors, choose chocolate instead!

You can also purchase something different such as popcorn, pretzels, fun pencils or stickers. The most memorable houses are not for the candy, but for the décor, costumes, or scary music playing as kids walk up to the door. Most visitors could care less what is being handed out when there is a moving skeleton surprise or furry spider!

D.I.E.T. #304

Buy one bag of Halloween candy, and plan something else for entertainment of your visitors. Place candy in the bowl you will hand it out from so you are prepared to give it all away. When the candy is gone, plan to have another item ready, or to turn out your lights.

October 31

It's the perfect day to focus on the color orange. Instead of trying to avoid candy, give yourself some easier directions. Orange foods, when they are naturally occurring, typically contain antioxidants and fiber. Beta carotene, the orange pigment found in plant foods, turns into Vitamin A in the body. Vitamin A is important in skin, soft tissue, and eye health, among its many other roles.

Pick something orange to eat today, or stretch yourself to eat orange at every meal. My favorite easy to find orange foods include carrots, orange peppers, cantaloupe, mangoes, sweet potatoes, and of course oranges! On Halloween, pumpkin is a sure bet for some beta carotene, but be careful to use 100% pumpkin without added sugar, or consume the actual squash itself, roasted in the oven.

D.I.E.T. #305

Cook something orange. Instead of focusing on what you shouldn't be eating today, focus on what you should be including.

November 1

By now, I'm sure you've realized that access is everything. This is especially true with unhealthy options. When there are unhealthy foods around, it is really hard to avoid them. I know it seems obvious, but you might need some ordering around to actually carrying out this suggestion. So, if you're listening, I am wearing my police hat and telling you, today is the perfect opportunity to kick temptations out of your house. Get to it!

Get rid of any extra Halloween goodies. Toss candy, unless you have kids who will keep their own small stash. Throw out cookies and other tempting items. Refuse the offer to take home leftovers from work or other gatherings. Give these items away to a candy collection, if there is one in your area. The goal for today is to accept the idea of wasting sweets. Throwing things away that will hurt you in the long run is not wasteful. In fact, if you don't, you'll be "waist-full!"

D.I.E.T. #306

Throw out extra candy. Right now!

November 2

Feeling comforted is a reason that many people choose to eat. The drive to feel secure often ends in a big meal of pasta, a giant bowl of ice cream, or an entire bag of chips. The problem with eating for comfort is that the foods we choose tend to be heavy, sugary, or fattening. When needing comfort, people continue to eat until the portion consumed is well beyond what is appropriate. Then, the cycle of needing to be comforted continues, with guilt as the precursor.

Instead of reaching for food, look to something else. On a fall night, a warm blanket is soothing, and provides the user with security. Children sleep with blankets for security and comfort, so why can't adults learn to reach for something besides food for comfort?

D.I.E.T. #307

Wrap up in a warm blanket. Even if you don't need comforting, consider that it is much harder to snack when wrapped up in a blanket!

November 3

If you've wiped down your counters, shined up your appliances and cleaned out your refrigerator, it is time to get organized! When you have things better arranged, it is less stressful to be in the kitchen, and you can be more efficient with prepping and cooking. Organization can seem daunting, so think about completing one project at a time. Working on one drawer in the kitchen is a great place to start.

If you have a cooking utensil or junk drawer in your kitchen, I suggest starting there. Purchase an adjustable divider or use shallow bins to hold items in place. Throw away melted spatulas or utensils that have lost their nonstick coating. If you'd rather, choose your most utilized items and place them in a jar style holder next to the stovetop.

D.I.E.T. #308

Organize a kitchen drawer. This will help keep you efficient in the kitchen, and might motivate you to spend more time cooking!

November 4

Improving your posture is a great way to relieve pain and increase energy, but you will have to practice! Improving posture is a major commitment, and it will require some consistent practice. If you've never focused on it, you likely have some work to do, so decide to make the commitment today. Every time you find yourself in a slouching position, repeat the following steps:

Straighten yourself in your chair, with your feet flat on the floor. Lift your chest up and drop your elbows and shoulders down. Pull your belly inward and imagine your abdominals hugging your spine to lift you taller. Breathe a few times in and out in this position. Repeat these steps at regular intervals or as often as you can remind yourself.

D.I.E.T. #309

Commit to your posture by sitting up tall as often as possible today. If needed, write yourself a note to remember to sit up straight!

November 5

One of the toughest challenges you can accept is to live in the moment. It might be confusing to understand exactly what that involves. As far as eating goes, it means you will have to think about what you are eating, how it tastes, what kind of experience you are having, and if you are getting satisfied. This might seem silly, but most people don't think about what, when, or how they are feeling when eating.

For today, make it a priority to think about how you are feeling and what you are experiencing when eating. Notice if you finish a meal that you don't really like, or if you keep eating a food when you are feeling full. Decide if what you are eating makes you feel good, and if you could stop a little bit sooner.

D.I.E.T. #310

Attempt to live in the moment during meals. Consider how much you are enjoying the food you are eating, and how satisfied you are becoming.

November 6

When it starts to get cold outside, it gets harder to stay motivated to exercise. To combat this decreased motivation, break out of your typical patterns. A walk outside might not be feasible, but a circuit workout set up around your house is a fun change to a routine. If you need more structure and direction, dust off an old workout video or purchase a new one.

Choose something that offers a heart rate increase for your effort. Anything that says "aerobics," "cross training", or "circuits" will likely keep your interest and get you breathing harder. Sometimes you can preview these online to see if you enjoy the exercise and don't mind the instructor! If you have enough space, recruit a friend or relative to try the video with you.

D.I.E.T. #311

Consider a workout video today. Depending on other exercise modes you are committed to, repeat the video at least once a week. As you get stronger, try the harder modifications that are almost always offered by the instructor.

November 7

When a person starts a food journal, they might discover that more calories are eaten between meals than at meals. Recording every little thing that is consumed is an eye opener to how much we graze. It is okay to spread out your eating, but be aware that when snacking, foods may not be as carefully selected.

Keeping food out of sight is a technique that seems obvious, but many people leave boxes of crackers or cookies in clear containers in plain view. These foods are just begging to be consumed mindlessly. To make our snacking more conscious, require the extra step of removing them from cupboards and pantries!

D.I.E.T. #312

Avoid putting snacks out between meals. Clear your kitchen surfaces of between-meal snacks. It's not the end of the world if you eat between meals, but adding a step to slow down the process is helpful in allowing more purposeful snacking.

November 8

The holidays are meant for sharing, loving, and celebrating. It feels good to give, and it reminds us of our blessings. Before the holidays arrive, schedule a time to serve food to those in need. Food banks and shelters tend to get a lot of help on the actual holiday itself, so consider giving your time sooner than that, when the average person is out shopping or celebrating with pre-holiday parties.

It is a beautiful reminder of the value of food when you see others who are grateful for a meal. You might enter into this project thinking you will serve the stereotypical homeless man. It can be quite surprising when you see the eyes of children light up when offered a hot meal.

D.I.E.T. #313

Volunteer to serve food to others. You will be providing them with food, but you will receive more than they do when you serve and give of your time.

November 9

If you ask me, the biggest challenge in life is finding balance. In an effort to find life balance, begin with an exercise that will help your muscles find physical balance. If you decide to continue with this exercise over time, you will notice your balance improving and your ability to add more to your routine.

Increasing your stability while standing can allow you to bring balance to your exercise, thereby preventing injuries and building strength in muscles that can otherwise be tough to train. Start building stability with a simple exercise of standing on one leg. Bend and raise your other knee up toward waist level and keep your standing leg straight. Place hands on hips or arms out to the side. Hold this position as long as possible, then switch legs and hold for the same amount of time.

D.I.E.T. #314

Practice balance today, by standing on one foot. When this becomes easier, close the eyes, or add ankle weights.

November 10

When eating carbohydrates, most people choose portions that are well beyond the recommended serving sizes. Eating fewer carbs can be a helpful strategy in weight management, blood sugar control, and in improving certain digestive symptoms. If you are trying to lower your intake, it is helpful to discover how many carbohydrates are present in the foods we choose to eat. Hint: they tend to add up quickly!

Try limiting your carbohydrates today. Notice if it is hard to do, if there seem to be carbs everywhere, or if it improves your energy level. Read labels, and recognize that breads, pasta, rice, fruit, dairy, beans, and starchy vegetables such as potatoes and corn are high in carbohydrate. Limit portions of these foods to one cup total at each meal. Focus on higher protein snacks and avoid juice and sugary beverages today.

D.I.E.T. #315

Go low carb today. Limit or avoid carbohydrates that you might typically choose, instead choosing lean proteins and non-starchy vegetables.

November 11

Getting ready to exercise doesn't just mean mentally preparing. It also means getting your body ready to take on more effort. Warming up the muscles can be thought of as warming up your car on a cold morning. If you don't allow your car a moment to get going, it won't run as well when you pull out of the driveway.

Give yourself at least three minutes of low intensity moving prior to exercising. This means moving, or dynamic stretches, or perhaps walking or jogging. Depending on your exercise of choice and your fitness level, a warm-up could be more or less intense. The goal is to ease into it, in order for your muscles to do their best work during exercise.

D.I.E.T. #316

Warm up prior to exercise. Get the most out of your workout by starting with a few moving stretches to loosen up.

November 12

Calories add up quickly, and some of the most calorically dense sources are sometimes overlooked. One of the best actions you can take when trying to improve your calorie intake is to limit or avoid alcohol. You don't have to do it cold turkey, and you likely don't have to give it up all together. However, giving up drinks is a great way to be healthier, especially for today.

Focusing on one thing at a time is meant to be simple, and today is no different. No alcohol. For most, this won't be extremely difficult, but for some, no drinking means skipping an evening glass of wine, or a beer with friends. It might feel like you're missing out on something, but remember that tomorrow you won't feel that way!

D.I.E.T. #317

Skip alcohol. If you don't drink now, consider it done, and pat yourself on the back for having a healthy habit already in place!

November 13

It is important to be realistic and specific when setting goals, while also creating strategies that will help you meet those goals. When it comes to snacking, being purposeful and thoughtful about food choices will help keep your body energized while maintaining a healthy weight.

To be specific with a snacking strategy is our challenge today, so start with the rule that all snacks have to come from the refrigerator. Why the fridge? There are certainly exceptions, but refrigerated foods are more likely fresh, whole choices. If you don't have much in your fridge, pick up some apples, carrots, yogurt, string cheese, or hard-boiled eggs to fill up in between meals. This strategy will help you consume extra nutrients and fiber today, while potentially lowering your total calorie intake.

D.I.E.T. #318

Limit snacks to foods found in the refrigerator. Specific and realistic goals are made easier with simple strategies such as eating fresh, whole foods.

November 14

When I was little, my grandmother taught me how to crochet, and as an adult, I learned how to knit. Though I don't think I can remember how to do either, I find that working with my hands, either by typing, sewing, or cleaning helps keep my mind occupied too.

Hobbies requiring your hands include playing musical instruments, gardening, woodworking, and participating in sports. Getting busy with your hands can keep you interested in the task at "hand," instead of what you are going to eat next. It's a way you can distract yourself with something constructive and enjoyable. Stress reduction through active hobbies, instead of food, will keep you feeling and looking healthier.

D.I.E.T. #319

Find a hobby to occupy your hands. Reach for that hobby when you are tempted to eat. Keep your hands busy to more easily avoid temptations!

November 15

If casseroles were an invention, the creator was a genius! Casseroles are always a welcome sight on our dinner table. They are comfort food at its best, and can include all of the necessary nutrients in one delicious package! Unfortunately, they can also be calorie-laden and full of unhealthy fats. The good news is that there are many modifications that can be made to easily improve your favorite casserole recipe.

Try swapping ingredients. Some of my favorite swaps include utilizing fat free, plain Greek yogurt for sour cream, or using low fat butter blends (not margarine), in place of real butter. Try pureed cottage cheese instead of ricotta, whole grain pastas, and consider extra vegetables to add volume. Sometimes you can even swap proteins, such as using ground chicken or turkey in place of beef. Top your casserole with lower fat cheeses, or use stronger flavored cheese so you can use less than normal.

D.I.E.T. #320

Experiment with a healthier version of a favorite casserole. You might like the healthier version better!

November 16

It might be a couple of weeks away, but Thanksgiving is near, and it takes careful planning to avoid having fourteen starches and not enough vegetables! Making a rough list of the main dishes, appetizers, sides, and desserts is helpful if you are hosting. If you are attending, think ahead to come up with a lighter, greener side dish to bring along.

If you normally make a heavy potato dish, consider utilizing riced cauliflower in place of some of the potatoes. If you are famous for your pumpkin pie, think about options such as a crust-less version or a vegan variety. Another option is to request to bring the green vegetable, and provide fresh green beans instead of casserole, or a mixed green salad with a light dressing. Thanksgiving doesn't have to set you back if you think ahead!

D.I.E.T. #321

Plan your Thanksgiving feast. A bit of pre-planning can make all the difference in how the holidays affect your health goals.

November 17

Intentions are great, but action is required to achieve goals. So, do something today that will prepare you for action! Write down a plan for exercise, including how you will be active for the next two weeks. Use a daily calendar or enter reminders into a smart phone or device.

When you record your exercise plan, be specific. Include two weeks of daily exercise goals. Enter a structured aerobic exercise into your calendar at least every other day, and strength training at least three times weekly. Fill in the rest of your plan with balance, stretching, yoga, meditation, and core strength. Make sure you add the approximate time of day you will workout, so you can prioritize your exercise. Don't forget to include a place to mark off your accomplishments each day.

D.I.E.T. #322

Write down your exercise plan for the next two weeks. Prioritize completion of your workouts by specifying times and modes of exercise.

November 18

Including more healthy fats is a simple goal for today. You'll feel fuller for longer, and provide your body with longer lasting energy. A great tasting, portable way to consume them is nut butter. We've discussed grinding your own, and different ways to include healthy fats, but today only focus on including or purchasing any type of nut butter.

If peanut butter isn't for you, you're ready to try something new or you're allergic, try almond, cashew, sunflower seed, or soy butters. There are many more options, so explore and try something different if you like. Keep in mind the serving size for healthy fat foods, which is one ounce. In nut butters, this equates to two tablespoons, or about as much as you'd see on a typical sandwich. Don't limit yourself to a sandwich though! Dip apples or celery, or spread on whole grain crackers for a filling snack.

D.I.E.T. #323

Enjoy nut butter. Explore the store for new varieties, and enjoy a new satisfying snack or addition to your meals.

November 19

As the holidays close in, I like to prepare my kitchen with a deep clean. It is important to me to use food safe cleansers and if I'm saving up for gifts, I love to utilize homemade cleaning tips. One of the best ingredients for cleaning a kitchen is likely already in your pantry—Vinegar!

Vinegar is a natural disinfectant and can clean a variety of surfaces. I like to use it on my kitchen floor, microwave, and glass surfaces. You might be thinking, "Her kitchen must stink!" Let me assure you that vinegar is not used at full strength! Dilute ½ cup distilled white vinegar in a half gallon of warm water for mopping the floor. Boil one cup of water with ¼ cup vinegar in the microwave until you notice steam on the door, then wipe away! Use equal parts vinegar and water to clean windows and other glass surfaces.

D.I.E.T. #324

Clean your kitchen with vinegar, or another home-made disinfectant. Don't use vinegar on porous surfaces like stone or granite countertops.

November 20

If you have a list with you at the grocery store, it is much easier to shop with intention. A few other tips that help prevent overbuying include shopping with a time limit, shopping after a meal, and limiting coupons to only those items you truly need.

Some people argue that being in a hurry creates temptation to simply throw things in the grocery cart without thinking. This can happen, so instead, try shopping a well thought out list with a time limit, such as by fitting your trip between activities. This prevents extra browsing and can keep you from making additional purchases. It is easy to get off course if you are hungry, so I suggest shopping after a meal, when you are less likely to buy things that are tempting to an empty stomach. Limiting coupon use to the items you truly need also keeps you organized in your trip.

D.I.E.T. #325

Stay on course with your holiday grocery shopping. Be efficient by purchasing off your list, staying within a time limit, and avoiding the store when hungry.

November 21

While buying gifts off wish lists can seem impersonal and uncreative, you are guaranteed to purchase something that the recipient wants or needs. On the flipside, remember that creating one isn't selfish or greedy, since there are likely people who will ask what you would like as a gift for the approaching holidays. People who ask what is on your list don't want to hear, "I don't know!"

What should you put on a wish list? Think about what would help you achieve better health. Some of my favorites gifts to give (*and* receive) are journals, fun water bottles and cups, kitchen tools, dishes, and exercise equipment. Workout clothes, spa gift cards, and yoga mats also top my list of favorites. If you've found a restaurant or meal delivery service that fits your health goals, request a gift card.

D.I.E.T. #326

Build a wish list full of things that will help you on your healthy journey. I've only suggested a few of my top choices!

November 22

It is common advice to save room for eating when you know you will be gathering for a meal. This makes sense, except for the chance that it could backfire as your stomach growls and you see all of the delicious options available! Depending on the gathering, it is typically best to have a high fiber snack ahead of time.

If you are trying to avoid overdoing it, have something that will lower your appetite, about one to two hours prior to the start of the event. Fiber helps to stave off cravings and hunger, and it is best consumed with a glass of water, to increase satiety even more. I suggest low calorie fiber containing foods such as raw vegetables, light popcorn, or a few whole grain seedy crackers.

D.I.E.T. #327

Fill up ahead of time. Aim to consume about five grams of fiber with at least eight ounces of water, about one or two hours prior to party time.

November 23

The sense of taste, of course, is the one that is primarily focused on when eating. There can be so much more to your experience if you use other senses as well!

Kids who have sensory problems with food are taught to smell, feel, and touch their food, instead of just looking and possibly tasting. Adults can do this too, to enhance satisfaction from eating. Today, notice how food feels in your mouth, the textures, and the different tastes that you may not have noticed before. Similarly, pay more attention to the smell of your food as well as the presentation of it.

D.I.E.T. #328

Use more of your senses today. You can enhance your sensory response to a meal, just by slowing down to pay closer attention. This can greatly impact your level of satisfaction and satiety.

November 24

In a season of thanks and grace, thinking about our blessings is important, but we may end up spending less time thinking about those less fortunate. While I know the holidays are about giving thanks, I need to remind myself not to forget about those who have less to be thankful for. Praying for them will remind you of your own abundances.

In general, thinking of others can remind us to be thankful. Praying for others opens the doors to grace in our own lives. Having a life focused on grace gives us freedom from things like addiction, lethargy, and apathy. It connects us to others, helps us value our health, and allows us to appreciate the ability to be physically active.

D.I.E.T. #329

Pray for someone. Notice how it feels to think more of others than of yourself, how it can change your perspective, and how it ultimately results in feelings of freedom and better health.

November 25

Learning to appreciate food for what it provides is important in your quest to select the best choices for your body. Being grateful in general, allows a more positive lifestyle because it affects the activities you choose, relationships you are involved in, and the way you value your time.

Everyone can be grateful for food, but being thankful for what it provides to us can help us see food as purposeful. Besides being thankful for food, remember other blessings such as the ability to be active and the ability to make your own choices. These also bring happiness, and have nothing to do with food. Being grateful for a body that functions well can bring us to exercise more often, and being thankful for family may encourage us to prioritize a home cooked meal to share together.

D.I.E.T. #330

Write down five things you are grateful for. This exercise will encourage you to stay positive and focused on the things you value most, including your health.

November 26

Most people like structure, but when traveling, it is hard to adhere to your regular schedule. When you leave your home environment, you have to adapt to a different routine. Keep this in mind when planning for the holidays. If you don't plan to travel, remember that your routine may change anyway with time off of work, social gatherings, or out of town visitors.

It is especially helpful to keep a journal of your goals, food intake, and exercise plan when your normal structure gets interrupted. Keep the journal in a place where you will see it daily, and continue to record what you are doing, even if it isn't in line with your goals.

D.I.E.T. #331

Stay on course when you leave home or travel for the holidays. Keep a journal and ask someone to help you stay accountable. If you are comfortable with it, let others know of your intentions.

November 27

Searching for warmth and comfort is more difficult in the winter. Finding it from heavy, warm meals is not as helpful as getting it from warm beverages such as tea or lemon water, hot showers or baths, and other indulgences. Many people struggle to eat healthy in the winter as they cozy up in baggy sweaters and sweatpants. Today, search for healthier ways to stay warm that are unrelated to food.

Building a fire outside or in, or turning one on is a great distraction, and also a way to quickly feel cozy! Watching a fire burn can be mesmerizing, and if you are cold or stressed, distracting yourself while warming up is especially helpful in calming down.

D.I.E.T. #332

Cozy up to a fire. Whether by campfire, fire pit, or fireplace, warmth can be calming. Just don't stand too close, and leave the marshmallows in the pantry!

November 28

It's been said that what doesn't kill you makes you stronger. It's certainly true that actions that feel impossible in the moment become easier with practice. Practicing hard things over and over creates a sense of ease and as a result, difficult tasks become achievable.

Picking something hard to achieve and taking mighty steps toward it is a great strategy. What you are capable of is probably not anything you can imagine today, so choose a goal that seems impossible in your near future. Then, determine a task to achieve today that you can achieve only with great effort. While working on that task, think about how it will be easier the next time you do it.

D.I.E.T. #333

Do something that seems really hard today. Remember that achieving it will make you stronger, and will take you toward your "impossible" goal!

November 29

Beans, beans the magical fruit, the more you eat the more you...! Due to their fiber and fermentation in the gut, legume types of beans such as black, pinto, and kidney cause gas. It is a good thing for your digestive tract, even though the symptoms might not feel that way! If you can tolerate them, beans are a great way to obtain fiber and are a balanced energy source of carbohydrate and protein. They also provide many B vitamins and minerals such as magnesium, iron, and phosphorus.

There are many ways to enjoy beans. Add them to soups, casseroles, tacos, or Sloppy Joes, enjoy them plain, or with a side dish of rice. If you eat a small portion, such as a half cup or less, you should be able to tolerate them. If not, you can try taking an enzyme such as galactosidase, or "Beano" prior to eating beans in a meal. The enzyme helps break down carbo-hydrates quicker, so they don't have time to ferment in the gut.

D.I.E.T. #334

Eat beans today. Try them on their own, in a side dish, or as a main course.

November 30

Habits are choices that when made over and over, eventually turn into lifestyles. When thinking about your health, you may have bad habits that are simply cycles that need to be broken. Disrupting these cycles help us disrupt the habits, thus "breaking" them.

Maybe you eat when you are stressed, and you are stressed when you come home from work. The cycle continues when you go to the pantry, dig into the pre dinner snacks, and feel better temporarily. Later, you feel worse, and ultimately, the cycle of being upset and stressed out is not broken, but continuous. This might not be one of your personal struggles, but searching for the cycles that are affecting your daily routine is a great step in breaking unhealthy habits.

D.I.E.T. #335

Look for cycles in your daily life. Determine which part of the routine you can change to disrupt the cycle, and you'll eventually break the habit.

December 1

Amid the chaos of holiday shopping, we tend to forget about taking care of ourselves. Today, think about what health goal you would choose if you could give it as a gift to yourself. Maybe it is better stress management, or a better energy level, or perhaps it is something more measurable like good lab results or a healthy weight. Or, pick a goal from my list of favorites, and commit to achieving it by the end of the month.

1. Improve your sleep by reading instead of watching television before bed.
2. Exercise in the morning hours for a better energy level later in the day.
3. Attend a yoga class at least once a week to better manage stress.
4. Eat at least 20 grams of protein for breakfast, to avoid afternoon cravings that can lead to weight gain.
5. Avoid fried foods to improve cholesterol levels and overall health.

D.I.E.T. #336

Pick a goal from my top five, and give yourself the gift of health.

December 2

Having more hours in the day has always been a dream of mine. Since I know it's never going to happen, the next best thing is to improve how I spend my time. When it comes to time, quality is better than quantity anyway!

Finding ways to spend time more efficiently is helpful, but finding activities that offer more enjoyment is important too. For example, multitasking a core workout while helping kids with homework is efficient, but spending time playing a game of tag with your kids might give you better returns. The same goes for food intake, remembering that improving the kinds of food you eat and your experiences around food will make a positive difference in your health.

D.I.E.T. #337

Notice what you are spending time on, and determine which activities will add health and wellness to your life. Focus on including activities and foods that enhance your quality of life, and reducing those that don't.

December 3

As a child, you may have disliked many foods because of their texture, flavor, or smell. Kids don't usually love vegetables, and they may also turn their noses up to strong tasting or unfamiliar foods. However, taste buds evolve, and many palates become more accepting with time.

For children, the "one taste" rule is very appropriate, as over time, a sample of a food can become more acceptable. Trying it over and over may allow you to lower your sensitivity to the food's unfamiliar texture and flavor. Similarly, if you don't like a food as an adult, give it another try. Try adding it to something, such as mushrooms in a casserole, or tomatoes on a pizza. You may be able to find more ways to add variety to your food intake.

D.I.E.T. #338

Try a healthy food you thought you didn't like, such as a particular vegetable or dairy product. Adult taste buds can change too!

December 4

Recording tips, making lists, and prioritizing goals are examples of how to maximize your success with the daily approach of D.I.E.T.S. 365. How do you remember it all day after day? If you have good note taking skills, you won't have to! If you haven't already, it is definitely helpful to take notes in this book. You will be reminded of strategies that work, and if you read the book more than once, you can reflect on your previous experiences.

As you read, record your thoughts, set goals, and make notes for days that inspire you the most. Dog-ear pages you would like to go back to, in order to measure your progress and consider practicing the strategy again. Using sticky bookmarks is another way to identify your favorite entries.

D.I.E.T. #339

Mark up this book! Take notes, fold corners of helpful pages, or use sticky bookmarks for entries you are inspired by. Then return to them over and over!

December 5

You may already have the tools in your kitchen to get creative with your cooking. It is easy to get stuck in a rut utilizing the stovetop to cook pasta, and the oven to bake frozen items, so let's get creative today! Think of a way to use your kitchen appliances differently.

Some suggestions include using a gas stovetop for roasting vegetables, as many online videos demonstrate. Use your oven to "bake" eggs, instead of using the stovetop to fry them. A greased muffin tin works great for this. Another suggestion is using a smaller appliance such as a waffle iron, to make pressed Panini style sandwiches. You can even use the microwave to steam chicken when you are crunched for time.

D.I.E.T. #340

Use a kitchen appliance in a different way. You'll stay home for more meals, fight food boredom, and have more ways to quickly prepare tasty, healthy choices!

December 6

It is always better to give than to receive. If you've volunteered or donated to a good cause, you understand this! The holiday season is a time when people in need are greatly saddened by their circumstances. The act of giving is uplifting to all involved, and can allow deep gratitude to be planted in the hearts of the giver and the receiver.

Look around and you will see giving trees, red kettles, blood donation mobiles, and opportunities to volunteer. If you don't have a lot of money to spend, it may be easier to give of your time. You will see delight in the eyes of the people you serve, no matter if you are offering a helping hand or a monetary donation.

D.I.E.T. #341

Select a charity and a way to donate. Food banks, shelters, and toy drives are all great ideas, but there are also red kettles to man, meals to cook, and blood banks in need.

December 7

It's a tempting time of year, and the tradition of cookie baking makes it harder! It is nearly impossible to avoid baking and it's fun to enjoy sweet treats this time of year. Go easy on yourself by enjoying in moderation and by experimenting with lighter recipes.

Now is the time to explore new recipes, so you can test them out prior to the holiday. If you have a cookie exchange coming up or a holiday gathering, search for ideas that are lighter. Recipes such as meringue style cookies, simple sugar cookies, and recipes that can utilize lightened ingredients are examples. Stronger flavors, such as molasses or ginger cookies often mean less sugary and fattening ingredients are needed.

D.I.E.T. #342

Bake a healthier cookie. If you simply can't make a different type, consider making smaller portions, using a half batch of dough for the same number of cookies.

December 8

If you ask me, snow is one of the prettiest things to see, but most annoying things to deal with. Depending on where you live, it could be the season to see a lot of white, but for today, avoid seeing it on your plate. White typically indicates food that has been stripped of its nutrients, protein, and fiber. What remains is primarily carbohydrates, sugars, and sodium.

There may be certain white foods that don't indicate "unhealthy," but it is safe to say that more color on your plate is healthier in general. Even though brown isn't much more exciting, it is healthier to eat whole grains versus processed. Brown rice, pasta, crackers, cereals, and bread products look healthier, and they are, as long as the word "whole" is indicated first on the ingredient label.

D.I.E.T. #343

Avoid the white stuff. Look to add color to your plate, but also read labels to consume only whole grains today.

December 9

Why did the tomato blush? Because he saw the salad dressing! Maybe this isn't the funniest joke ever, but finding a way to laugh through stressful times is therapeutic. Not surprisingly, studies show that laughter helps a person live a longer, better quality life. You don't have to read joke books, but even a quick online search of funny jokes or videos is a great way to lighten up!

Watching a comedy or recorded show while you walk on the treadmill is a sure way to reduce stress. Going to bed earlier is a healthy behavior to work on, so if late night television makes you laugh, record an episode. Then, watch it at a better time of day. Remember, laughter burns calories too!

D.I.E.T. #344

Laugh several times today. If you aren't around funny people, bring yourself to laughter by reading, listening, or watching something entertaining.

December 10

It takes a very strong commitment to record your food intake accurately and completely. The first step is to have a place to write down what you are eating. Designate a notebook, device, or other place to document meals, amounts, and other details. To get started, use this page to write down *today's* food intake. If you read this page a second or third time, you can reflect on how your patterns have changed.

Write down everything, and don't judge yourself. This is a page that encourages you to reflect and then move forward!

D.I.E.T. #345

Keep food record notes here.

December 11

Reciprocation doesn't have to mean doing exactly what someone does for you. It means returning a favor in one of many ways. In my life, my true friends reciprocate and appreciate. Doing people favors without expecting reciprocation is also important. Today, offer help to someone who deserves your attention.

Remember a good deed that was done for you recently, and make it a point to recognize that person today. Think about people you may take for granted, such as coaches, teachers, mentors, or neighbors. It doesn't have to cost you a thing. Even saying, "Hey, I owe you one" counts, as long as you follow through!

D.I.E.T. #346

Reciprocate. Returning a favor allows more good fortune to come your way. Notice those who help you, and look for opportunities to help them in return.

December 12

Lean, toned legs might not be your focus in a season of jeans and sweat pants, but it's important to get started on your goals early! Even if your legs are already lean and toned, you need to protect your back from movements that cause injury if your legs aren't also strong.

Lifting with your legs will protect your back from overworking. How do you lift with your legs? Whenever you pick something up from the floor, bend at your knees, not your waist. Pull your belly inward and breathe out as you lift. If you already know this technique, do it all day, along with some extra squat exercises. If it is new to you, practice!

D.I.E.T. #347

Lift with your legs. Every time you pick something up from lower than knee level, practice bending your knees, and pull your belly button inward. The more you do this, the more natural it will become.

December 13

A lot of healthy goals include eating more vegetables, but today, the focus is to eat them first thing in the morning. That way, you're off to a great start on increasing your total intake. Vegetables might not sound good, and they may be difficult to incorporate at breakfast, so here are a few ideas to start with.

Scramble eggs with chopped peppers, onions or mushrooms, and top with salsa if you like. If you like eggs on a sandwich, top them with sautéed spinach or kale and serve on a whole grain bun or wrap. Try a sweet potato topped with cinnamon for breakfast! Use riced cauliflower and/or broccoli in a crust for a lightened quiche. One of my favorite swaps is to spread avocado on whole grain toast instead of butter (ok, an avocado is actually a fruit!)

D.I.E.T. #348

Have vegetables for breakfast. It seems challenging, but with a little planning ahead, you've got this!

December 14

There are likely shelters in your area that provide a hot meal to a family in crisis. It may be due to an accident, violence, or death, but the people served by these shelters are traumatized and hurting. While a homeless shelter is a great place to offer your time, a crisis center will typically accept homemade meals, snacks, premade meals, blankets and personal items.

Make arrangements to bring food or other items to a place in need, and determine what you will prepare. You may want to call ahead so you can bring the supplies that are most depleted. This type of service might be even more rewarding than past volunteering experiences, as you will offer your time and resources to someone in an urgent situation.

D.I.E.T. #349

Plan to provide a meal to a crisis center or emergency shelter. If food is not accepted, blankets and toys are often appreciated.

December 15

Most people think their dance skills are better than they actually are! Does it really matter? No matter your skills, do it for all the benefits. Dancing makes a person feel good, physically and mentally. It lightens moods and makes people smile, or maybe laugh! Depending on the intensity, dancing can burn a lot of calories too.

More than for the calories, dance today to improve your mood and reduce stress. Even if you don't feel stressed, laughing and smiling more will improve your quality of life. You don't need a dancing partner, but it might be better if you close the shades and get down in the privacy of your own home! In any case, practice your favorite moves for at least ten minutes today.

D.I.E.T. #350

Dance however you want to, even if you don't have all the moves! If you do it to burn calories or reduce stress, it doesn't matter. Just get grooving. Dancing is good for your health!

December 16

When gathering for holidays, it is easy to let food be the focus. Providing appetizers ahead of time helps everyone come together while the finishing touches are put on the meal. Appetizers, however, can be the easiest place to make mistakes. Cheesy, fattening, calorie-laden foods are typical choices, and are so deliciously tempting! You can better avoid this and set an example for those around you, by providing a lighter option.

Select vegetable based appetizers, avoid heavy dips, and provide single-bite choices. Something as delicious as stuffed mushrooms is an excellent example. If you choose to create a dip, use ingredients such as Greek yogurt, cucumbers, garlic, and lemon juice to create Tzatziki, or make a homemade hummus with chickpeas or white beans. Spread dips on crackers ahead of time and add garnish to provide a single bite choice.

D.I.E.T. #351

Create a healthy appetizer. Do this with vegetable based items, light ingredients, and single bite servings.

December 17

Have you ever used cheesecloth? If you haven't it might sound weird, but trust me, it is a nice tool to have on hand. Traditionally, it is used to strain liquids off the curds when making cheese, hence the name! However, this time of year you might use it to strain stocks for gravy, or to dust cookies with powdered sugar, which is a great swap for frosting those healthier Christmas cookies.

Place cheesecloth in a strainer to catch solids, or place it over a mason jar filled with powdered sugar, then tighten with the metal ring. It's an instant shaker! You can also use it for my favorite purpose, which is to wring out steamed vegetables before ricing them for crusts or other recipes. If you are ambitious, cheesecloth is also used in straining homemade yogurt, and in making tofu.

D.I.E.T. #352

Buy something weird at the store, such as cheesecloth. It's cheap, and it might just come in handy.

December 18

Creating a festive meal to share with others is gratifying, and helps in stirring up the holiday spirit. This year, decide on a menu and a guest list, and include someone you wouldn't normally think to invite. One year, we had a friend of the family attend our holiday meal. As a single man without family nearby, Josh expressed gratitude for including him.

Keep the menu simple and healthy. A small roasted turkey or Cornish hen, roasted sweet potatoes, a large green salad, and whole grain dinner rolls come to mind, but get creative if you like. Ask your guests to bring an appetizer so you won't have it around while you are cooking. As far as dessert, an after dinner sorbet or fruit cups with a bit of whipped topping are refreshing.

D.I.E.T. #353

Invite someone over for a holiday meal. Remember the golden rule; "treat others the way you want to be treated." It feels good to help others!

December 19

When my grandfathers were alive, my dad used to enjoy eating pickled herring with them around the holidays. While I found it pretty repulsive, there are some benefits I wasn't thinking of at the time! Now that my father continues to eat it, I can praise him for doing something good for his health.

While high in sodium, pickled foods like vegetables, and healthy fat foods such as herring, can provide nutrients, fiber and healthy fat in a salty and satisfying snack. Some of my favorites for health include herring for omega 3 fats, and green beans or asparagus for fiber. Fermented foods are a subcategory of pickled foods, but are pickled by a different process. Choosing fermented foods by looking for "live active cultures" on the label provides the added benefit of maintaining healthy gut flora.

D.I.E.T. #354

Eat something pickled. Better yet, choose a pickled and fermented food such as kimchi, cultured cheeses, or sauerkraut.

December 20

Being open and honest is hard, and can be humbling. It is also the reason so many people don't achieve goals. Declaring to yourself that you have made mistakes is the first step to working through those mistakes and living a changed lifestyle.

Perhaps you have denied a food addiction or eating disorder. It could be helpful to admit major stressors like this, so the proper steps to rehabilitate can be taken. Maybe your confession is not that big, but you fail to be honest on food records, or you don't do the workout that was prescribed for you. In order to get motivated to achieve these goals consistently, you must admit you aren't doing them well, and get help in working around your obstacles.

D.I.E.T. #355

Come clean with yourself or with someone else. It could be something simple, or maybe something major that is hard, but important to admit.

December 21

Speeding it up can be helpful in the holiday season, and all year round. Whether it is getting your grocery shopping done, getting work projects wrapped up, traveling, or wrapping gifts, it is always nice to speed up the process. Getting more done in a shorter period of time always feels productive. Today, consider accelerating your workouts without rushing.

It's not about being impatient or hurrying through things, but instead thinking about picking up your pace or cadence. In cycling, cadence is the rate at which the pedals rotate, and in running, cadence is the rate at which your legs turnover. Increasing that rate will make you faster, but your focus will be on pushing your legs instead of rushing your speed.

D.I.E.T. #356

Increase your cadence in all of your daily activities. This time of year, everyone is short on time, so think about acceleration today.

December 22

This time of year, you may be spending lots of time in the kitchen. Maybe you are taking some time off of work, or perhaps you are doing some holiday cooking and baking. Make the most of your kitchen today by doing a few counter top exercises. These will get your mind off munching, and will give you a little energy boost too.

My two favorites are counter push-ups and triceps dips, but stretching the shoulders and back are other ways to relax right in the kitchen. Place your hands on the counter, step your feet away so your arms are stretched out straight, and bend at the waist. Step back so that your chest can fold closer to your thighs. Try to keep your legs straight, then step back so your arms remain as straight as possible. Ideally, your back should end up parallel to the floor, keeping your tummy pulled in. Your head should hang weightless between your arms.

D.I.E.T. #357

Do counter top exercises. The counter stretch above is a great release for shoulder and neck tension, and is also a deep stretch for the back of the legs.

December 23

Calorie unawareness is a big problem. Being naïve to how much you are consuming is dangerous to your health. For most, carbohydrates are easy to overeat because they aren't very filling when consumed as proper portions. Carbs have a lot of calories relative to their nutritional value. Choosing foods with fewer calories and more nutrients is the way to go, so what should you eat instead of all those carbs?

Replace bread products at dinner with extra protein and veggies, which offer you a much bigger bang for your calorie. Examples include wrapping meats in lettuce instead of serving buns, stuffing peppers with ground meats, and eating eggs over spinach instead of toast. Even a cauliflower crust pizza fits into this rule. Eating your protein with veggies will allow you to stay fuller for longer.

D.I.E.T. #358

Instead of bread, use vegetables to serve your protein. You'll end up with more vitamins and fiber, but fewer calories!

December 24

Getting rid of extra desserts is simple when you believe in Santa, since you can set them out and they will disappear by morning! If you are past the point of believing, you can still put an end-date on your goodies. Today is the day to enjoy in moderation, save any you might need for entertaining tomorrow, and discard of the rest!

Why discard of them before the holidays are over? It is most helpful to stay in the right frame of mind by eliminating temptation and enjoying the beauty of the season in ways other than eating. Discard of sweets and appreciate other comforts such as holiday music, a religious service, or a warm cup of tea.

D.I.E.T. #359

Santa Claus can be helpful this time of year, even if you don't believe in him. Put leftover desserts out tonight; then ask someone else to make them disappear. You won't need the extras tomorrow!

December 25

Whether or not you are Christian, today's focus is love. Spreading and receiving love requires a grateful heart, so today, make sure you are appreciating others and showing your true love to those around you. If you can appreciate what love can achieve, you will be more wiling to continue to offer it.

Today, show someone around you an act of love. Presents are great, but they don't count for this D.I.E.T.! You must speak and show love to achieve your goal today. Tell someone *why* you love him or her, and be specific about it. If you'd rather show the act, remember that presents don't count. Show them physically with hugs, offer to spend time doing something special with that person, or talk about your favorite memories together.

D.I.E.T. #360

Show love. Today, make this task a priority by making it intentional.

December 26

If you've put yourself on a budget before, you know that eating out and buying processed foods is expensive. If you've ever been on a calorie-restricted diet, you've budgeted calories as well. There are certain snacks and foods that fit into a calorie budget easier, and a few snacks that cost so little in calories, they are considered "freebies."

Create your own list of freebies, and you can fill up with fewer calories. To be considered for the list, a free food must contain 20 or fewer calories and no more than 5 grams of carbohydrate. Raw vegetables are free, and anything non-starchy goes! If veggies don't cut it, try one to two cups of light popcorn, a ½ cup serving of berries, or a ½ cup sugar free Jell-O. You can even find frozen fruit bars that come in close enough to "free."

D.I.E.T. #361

Buy and choose snacks from your own freebie list. Enjoy these as often as you like.

December 27

Repeat a mantra during exercise to help you dominate your workout today. Repeating a positive message over and over may sound cheesy, but it works. Talking yourself into completing something difficult is a sure way to get it done.

Realize that the real work is what allows you to move forward. The work that makes you sore, and maybe cry, the work that makes you sweat, and that you don't think you can finish. That work is what will move you ahead and help you reach your goals. Everything gets easier next time, which is another great catchphrase to help keep motivated through the last few minutes or last few repetitions.

D.I.E.T. #362

Say I AM enough; I CAN do this; I WILL do this, as you complete your workout. Remind yourself that these efforts will allow you to do more in your next workout. If it's challenging, it's progress!

December 28

Carbohydrates aren't the enemy, but most people eat too many of them. A balanced diet for most active people should contain around 40-50 percent of calories from carbohydrate. This equates to about 200 grams of carb for a person eating 1,800 calories. It might seem like a lot, but it adds up quickly. Today, turn your attention to carbohydrate and record how many grams you eat without altering your patterns.

Ideally, a person would spread calories evenly throughout the day, and perhaps have more of the allotted carb earlier in the day versus later. In an ideal world, a person might consume 45 grams of carbohydrate at breakfast, lunch, and dinner, and about 30 grams at a mid morning and midafternoon snack.

D.I.E.T. #363

Count carbohydrate grams today. Note your patterns, total intake, and how food is spread through the day. Think about how you could improve your balance tomorrow.

December 29

Back pain is a the worst. I know because I have a lot of hardware taking up space around my spine. There are a lot of painful issues that can arise during the night, and it is no fun to wake up stiff and sore. Besides taking an anti-inflammatory, there are many other ways to prevent physical pain during sleep.

Sleeping with a pillow between my knees is something I've done since having back surgery in 2004. While I have to wake up to roll over, it is worth the reduction in lower back pain. Keeping a pillow in between the legs provides better alignment of the hips and spine, and can offer relief from knee pain as well.

D.I.E.T. #364

Try sleeping with a pillow between your knees, even if you don't have back pain. If you already do this, consider trying a longer body pillow.

December 30

The New Year is upon us, and there are many great deals to be had. Besides after- Christmas shopping, consider seeking out a gym that may be offering free trials or free classes to kick start the New Year. Many of these facilities actually offer these year round, but checking them out today is a simple step to get your New Year's goals rolling.

Even if you already belong to a gym, trying out other facilities can offer you a change of pace and perhaps challenge you in a method you haven't tried before. Cross training gyms, Barre or yoga studios, mixed martial arts, spinning and Pilates are just examples. If you are uncomfortable trying a new place, find a friend or family member who will do it with you.

D.I.E.T. #365

Try a gym that offers a free visit or free trial class. Even if you don't join, it's great to challenge your muscles in a new way.

December 31

When you are prepared, everything is easier. Planning a long-term goal a year in advance is great, but getting that goal accomplished takes everyday action. On New Year's Eve, so many people announce big goals for the next year, but today, focus on your goals for tomorrow. Having a vision for what tomorrow will hold is smart because you will prioritize your health and be determined to get things accomplished.

For example, if you have a plan to exercise, you will be less likely to make heavy food choices or drink alcohol the night before. When you have a plan to eat at home, you will prioritize getting to the store to get your ingredients. If your plan is to watch football, make a separate plan to be active prior to the game.

D.I.E.T. #366

Make a plan for tomorrow. It doesn't have to be complicated, but make sure it aligns with your goals for next year. You'll be off to a great start!

Beyond the First Year

Now that you've completed your readings for the year, continue your journey by returning to any bookmarked pages. Read through your notes and reflect on all you have achieved. Notice pages that are dog-eared and decide if you are still working on certain strategies.

If you decide to read *D.I.E.T.S. 365* a second time, you will notice that its challenges can serve you in new ways. Your baseline is likely healthier, so the strategies may remind you of the progress you have made. Even though you've made progress, there will likely be certain days that remain difficult. The point of reading a second or third time is to encourage continuous improvement.

Another way to utilize the book is to invite others to read, and take on these challenges alongside you. Start a book club that incorporates healthy goal setting, and offers that sense of community and group support. There are many ways to share with others, and continue to benefit from *D.I.E.T.S. 365*, even after the first year.

57382532R00204

Made in the USA
Columbia, SC
08 May 2019